HERO

12 Weeks to SUPERHERO FIT

MAKER

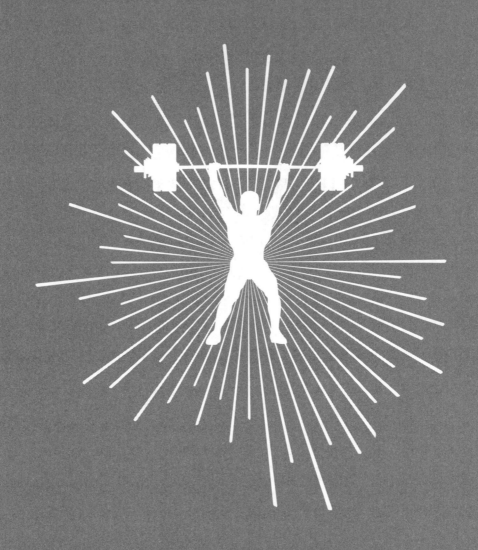

HERO

12 Weeks to SUPERHERO FIT

MAKER

A HOLLYWOOD TRAINER'S
REAL GUIDE TO GETTING THE BODY
YOU'VE ALWAYS WANTED

DUFFY GAVER

St. Martin's Griffin
New York

First published in the United States by St. Martin's Griffin, an imprint of
St. Martin's Publishing Group

HERO MAKER: 12 WEEKS TO SUPERHERO FIT. Copyright © 2020 by James Duffy Gaver. All rights
reserved. Printed in the United States of America. For information, address
St. Martin's Publishing Group, 120 Broadway, New York, NY 10271.

www.stmartins.com

Design by Susan Walsh

Library of Congress Cataloging-in-Publication Data

Names: Gaver, Duffy, author.
Title: Hero maker : 12 weeks to superhero fit : a Hollywood trainer's real
    guide to getting the body you've always wanted / Duffy Gaver.
Description: First edition. | New York : St. Martin's Griffin, 2020. |
    Includes index.
Identifiers: LCCN 2019048699 | ISBN 9781250096630 (hardcover) | ISBN
    9781250096647 (ebook)
Subjects: LCSH: Physical fitness. | Exercise.
Classification: LCC GV481 .G38 2020 | DDC 613.7—dc23
LC record available at https://lccn.loc.gov/2019048699

Our books may be purchased in bulk for promotional, educational, or business use.
Please contact your local bookseller or the Macmillan Corporate and Premium Sales Department
at 1-800-221-7945, extension 5442, or by email at MacmillanSpecialMarkets@macmillan.com.

First Edition: April 2020

10 9 8 7 6 5 4 3 2 1

For my son Jack—why be good when you can be great

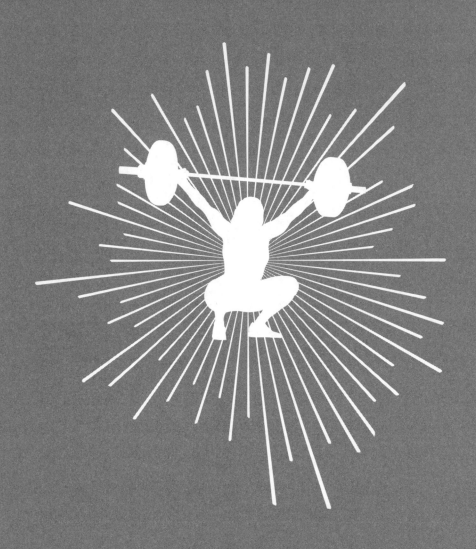

Contents

HERO

12 Weeks to SUPERHERO FIT

MAKER

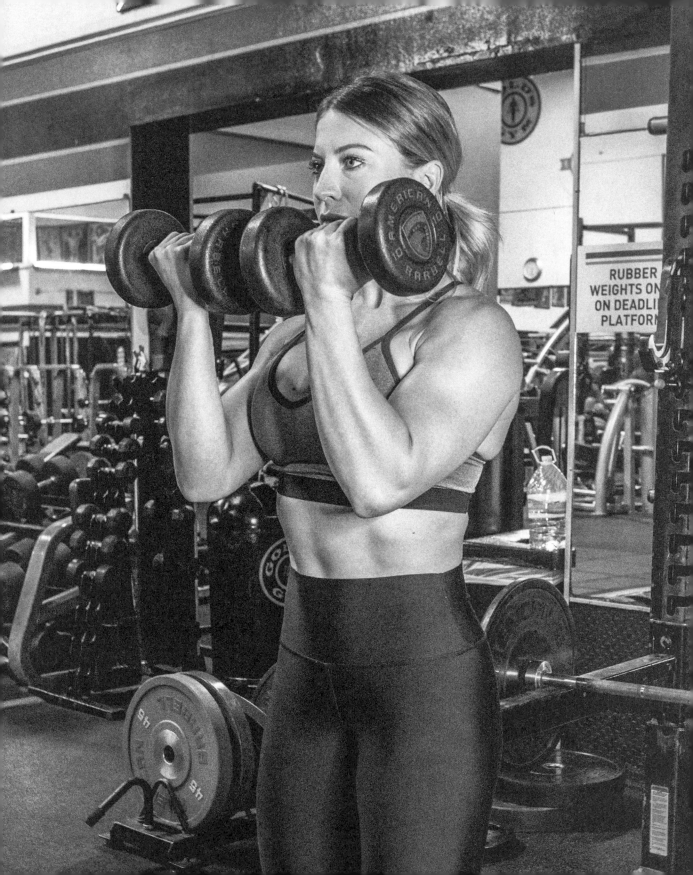

Introduction

Y ou've seen *Troy*, *Spider-Man*, *Guardians of the Galaxy*, *Thor*, *The Avengers*. You love the movies and you want to look like the actors who portray your favorite heroes. You probably think they are blessed with great genetics. Maybe they are. Or maybe you're convinced they just look that way because that's how actors look. Well, that's not entirely true. Every single one of them has worked their butt off to have the body that they have. That's the genetics of hard work.

Is it for you? Can you look like Chris Hemsworth, Scarlett Johansson, or Chris Pratt? I don't know. What I do know is what works—what's real and what isn't.

Let's start with this. How bad do you want it? You're holding this book. You picked it up. You bought it for a reason. If that reason is you just want to see what magic trick I have to offer, you've come to the wrong place. I'm not a magician. I don't have a magic formula. I'm not that guy.

To get a great body, you need to be ready to move fitness to the top of your priorities. You've got to be willing to do everything. And it's work. No part of this should be easy. If it was easy, everyone would look amazing.

What it all comes down to is you.

FITNESS STARTS WITH . . . *YOU.*

That's the only answer. There's no quick fix. You've got to get comfortable with how this really takes place. And you know what, if this all seems too daunting to you and you want to quit, then quit now. Save yourself the money. I won't be offended. You won't be offended. Or you can step up, be your own hero. See how this works?

And be ready to give it everything you have. As I always say to my clients, if you want to look amazing, you have to train amazing, you have to eat amazing, and you have to sleep amazing. If you're doing all of that, you are going to see great results.

Yes, it means sweating it out in the gym, your basement, or wherever. It also means being really disciplined about your diet. You've got to say no to that cocktail you want to drink, no to the doughnut, and no to going out with your friends tonight because you need to train hard tomorrow morning and you need to be well-rested.

The A-listers that I work with do all of these things to look the way they do. They get hired for a reason. It's not just their looks or their résumé. I've worked with everyone from Tobey Maguire for his role as Spider-Man to Scarlett Johansson as Black Widow to Chris Hemsworth for his role as Thor. Chris Pratt, too, for Star-Lord—his transformation was stunning. I could give you an endless list of major stars that I've crossed paths with. And the studios come to me because I know what I'm doing. They send stars to me who are serious about getting things done. They don't hire actors and actresses lightly. Not when you have $200 million riding on a film. There's a lot of pressure on you with that, so the stars take it seriously. When you know your body is going to be up on a seventy-foot screen and your shirt is going to be off or whatever they have you doing, you are going to show up. You are not going to quit. You're going to give it everything you have. Your entire career depends on it.

So if you're looking to lose weight or improve your fitness or simply get yourself moving again—yeah, I can help you. But first you've got to be honest with yourself. I talk to my clients about this all the time. You've got to have realistic goals. If you want to be lean and you weigh three hundred pounds, stop trying to be lean for the moment. Start by trying to lose some weight. If you're trying to be huge and you're built like a pencil, I have news for you: try packing on a little muscle mass at a time. You may never get that big. But start by improving where you are, and see if you can get there over time. Rushing to get there won't get you there.

Your goals need to be *real,* as in realistic. They need to be concise, not all over the place.

There is no shortcut to get where you want to go.

Let me repeat that: *no shortcut.*

When I was eighteen years old, I was going nowhere with my life. I was hanging out with the wrong people and going in the wrong direction. So my mom and my sister sat me down and we talked. I enlisted in the Marines after that. When I got to the Marines, at the rifle range during requalifying, a friend recommended I try out for STA (Surveillance and Target Acquisition) platoon and become a sniper. I was fortunate enough to be able to do that. It taught me a lot—determining who is a threat and who is not requires you to be sharp. They train you to do that—you're not born that way. And it takes years.

Overseas as a Marine, I spent some time working in conjunction with the Navy SEALs, so I decided to become one. This was not easy, but it was an important part of my life. I value my military training; it has helped define me as a person. It enables me to do my job well. I like to cut through the crap. I like to boil things down to what they really are. I get that from my training. In the military, you are taught to be more than you think are. If you have any doubt, you need to wipe that right out.

It's the same with your health or your body composition. You need to discard any preconceived notions you have. Wipe the slate clean. Start from the beginning. As if this is your first time.

Here's one of my favorite stories. I once sat on the beach after a long run with a woman who told me she was not the type of person that I trained, that she was different. As if some of us are born athletes and others are not. I understood what she was getting at, but I wanted to show how her thinking (her mental approach to being fit) was holding her back. I sat down next to her and I said, "That's your leg right there." I had her touch her leg. I said, "Those are your quads and those are my quads. They're exactly the same. My muscles are built out of the same tissues as yours are. They connect to all the same spots and do all the same things. The only difference is that I take mine out. You haven't done that, but now you will." She had to change her point of view, and she did. Now you start to see where this book, including my guidance and philosophy, is secondary to your mindset. Are you ready to get to work?

People always have these preconceived notions that they need to rid themselves of. If someone says to me, "I'm fat and big-boned," I might respond: "That may be what you think, but you're not thinking about your frame and how much muscle you might be able to pack onto your body." Or if someone says to me, "Look, I'm rail-thin, I'll never be big," I might say, "Okay, if that's true, what about how shredded you could get? Have you considered that?"

Instead of thinking about body types in negative terms, think about them positively. Which way do you think you are going to accomplish more?

You want to get shredded or get ripped? You want to lose weight? You want to be more than you are? Be better? Then you have to start by making things right in your head.

Fitness starts with one thing and one thing only: the decision to get fit.

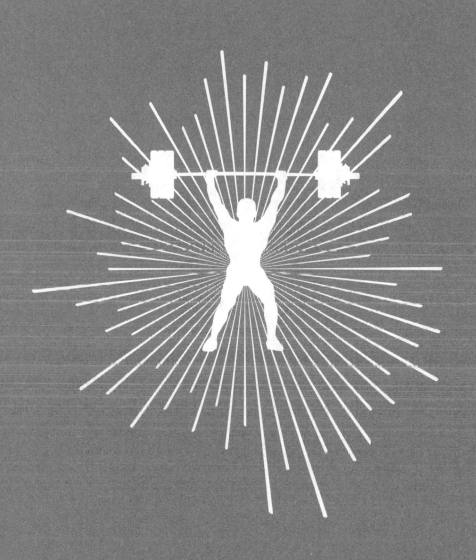

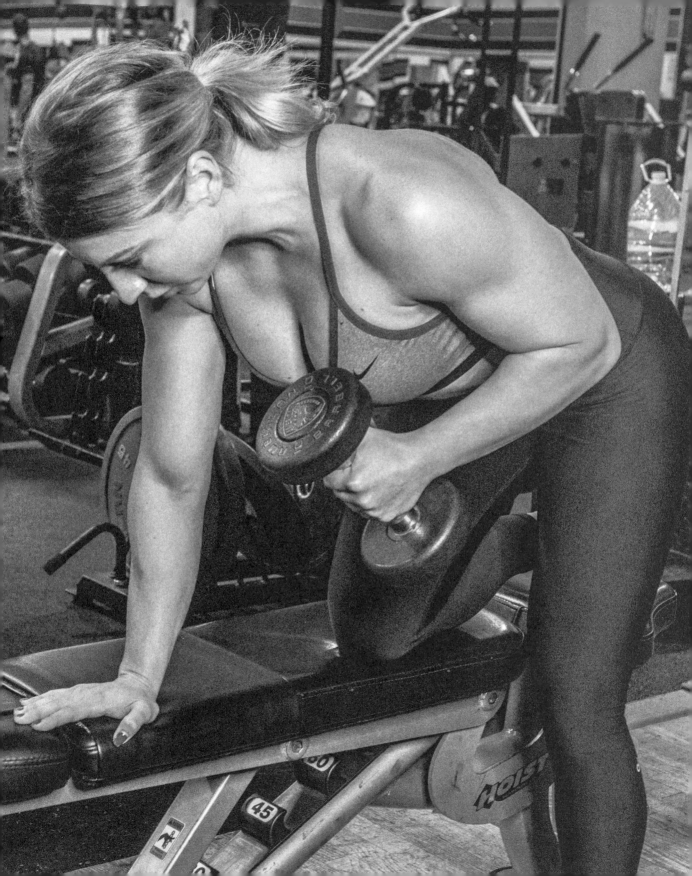

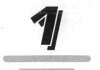

The Human Body Is Not New

The only easy day was yesterday.
—**Navy SEAL saying**

THE FITNESS INDUSTRY IS HURTING YOU

Over the last fifty plus years, the business of fitness has gone from being a cottage industry to a multibillion-dollar corporate behemoth, and a lot has gotten lost along the way. A corporate behemoth doesn't care about you. Those who run such companies have no interest in getting you fit or fixing you. They might say that they do, but their ultimate goal is to sell you stuff and to keep making money off of you. The goal of those in this business, like any other business, is to turn a profit. If they can sell you a new workout and make money from you, then they will sell you a new workout. And social media has only exacerbated the problem by giving a voice to fitness influencers who may not necessarily know what they are doing.

These companies get you because everybody wants to look great. They know that. They know everything they need to do to get you to buy their product or subscribe to their method. They want you to think that you can't do this without them. For example, you're in the mall and you see a store pushing protein powder. In the store window is a giant ad featuring some clean-shaved, super-ripped guy posing shirtless, holding up the "best-tasting protein powder the world has ever seen." Do you think that guy got ripped using that powder? He didn't. Chances are he doesn't even use that product. He's just a model getting paid to say, "Hey, if you use this, you can look like me, too." Maybe in that same store window (or maybe in an ad in a magazine) there's a photo of a woman in a tight-fitting outfit, with ripped arms and a curvy body, promoting the latest thermogenic supplement. Same thing. Do you think she uses that product? No. But the company that makes that product sure wants you to associate their product with that woman. That's how they get you.

The people you see in the ads for the products; they're on testosterone, decabolin, winstrol. This is the lie that gets sold to you. Don't fall for it.

I've been in this business many years. You can't look the way these people look using the products that they promote. I'm sorry, but that's garbage.

It's made up. It's not real.

I wish I had a magic pill for you. I really do. I could be a millionaire many times over if I actually had the magic pill, but it doesn't exist. What does exist are companies that make millions of dollars trying to make you think or believe that they do have a magic pill. Think about it. Diet trends are all over the place. One company tells you to try a cabbage diet, another the banana diet; some push gluten free or carb free. Whatever, it's all the same. Take this pack of pills in the morning, this pack at noon, and another pack before bed. And don't forget your predigested protein to build muscle. Here's your thermogenic pack to boost your metabolism, because most of the calories you're taking in with all of your nonstop protein drinks create no thermogenic effect on their own.

When you take all this stuff, you are actually doing more harm to yourself and to your progress than you are even aware of. It's like watching someone smoke weed to chill, do coke to get up, then drown himself in booze to calm down—it's not going to go well for you.

The companies push supplements at you. That's what they are there for—to remind you that you can't do this without them. Then the gyms or studios push their classes and instructors at you, whether you show up or not. How about the athletic wear companies? They're part of this, too. They push their new outfits with the latest, greatest scientific tech behind them. They push sneakers that will help you perform better. Ask yourself this: Does a pair of sneakers actually make you run faster? *But all the great athletes use this sneaker to be who they are.* Sound familiar? It's part of a marketing campaign. And none of these things that I've mentioned have anything to do with being fit.

Back in the day when people used to go for a run, they just called a buddy up: "Hey, man, you want to go run?" You went out, ran, and enjoyed yourself. You didn't invest time in finding the perfect running outfit or in obsessing over what kinds of shocks or specific foams were in your shoes. How did someone go for a run back in the day without that? How? My buddy Randy in the Marine Corps used to take tremendous pride in wearing the oldest, shittiest pair of Converse high-tops he could find and then smoking everybody when we went for our runs.

You tell me. Do you need products to become fit?

No.

If I now tell you that American obesity and type 2 diabetes are at the highest point they have ever been in history—keep in mind, this is with all the latest technology, all the extensive medical knowledge, all the best supplements, and all the greatest gyms and home gyms that are out there—what does this tell you? (According to the World Health Organization, worldwide obesity has nearly tripled since 1975. In the United States alone, the Centers for Disease Control and Prevention (CDC) reports that between 2015 and 2016, 93.3 million adults were obese, and obesity-related conditions such as heart disease, stroke, type 2 diabetes, and certain types of cancer were the leading cause of death—and yet all of this is preventable.) Think about it. Fifty years ago, people were healthier than they are today. How is that possible with everything you have available?

The simple truth is the fitness industry is not focused on getting people healthy. Instead it is built on making money and perpetuating false promises. The world has gotten very complicated over the years. There's a lot of misinformation (or disinformation) to sift through.

Well, let me make it easy for you. Let me uncomplicate it.

In 1965, Larry Scott became the first man to win Mr. Olympia. When he was in training, Hammer Strength machines didn't exist. Supplement companies weren't there to help him. He didn't have university studies to reveal what the most effective angle on a bench press was to increase muscle mass. And yet he looked as good as anyone has.

In 1954, Roger Bannister ran the first four-minute mile in human history. The first four-minute mile! That's a tremendous feat. Nike running shoes didn't exist. Machines that measured the length of Bannister's stride and the impact his foot made when it hit the ground weren't available. He was a runner. He ran. He ran his ass off.

In 1977, Bruce Wilhelm became the first World's Strongest Man. There were no established gyms or training methods to do what he did—much of the equipment that exists today didn't exist then—and yet he won the inaugural World's Strongest Man competition. He beat out other people to get there. Imagine that? He worked hard to beat those competing against him.

So again, what does all of this tell you?

It tells you that you don't need the supplements, the fancy machinery, the trendiest workout, or the latest gym outfit to get you pumped. What you need to do is get your ass to the next workout and save yourself the money that you would have wasted. Fitness is like a bank account. If you put in $100 day in and day out, then one day you get to have that million-dollar body you wanted. But if you're tossing in $100 bills here and there, $50 some days, loose change on occasion, then that's what you are going to get—not your million-dollar best but a lesser version.

Ask marathon runners how they do what they do. They don't run a whole marathon first thing; they run a mile and then another one and then another. If you keep that up for 26.2 miles, you've got a marathon.

If you're Eliud Kipchoge, you've done it in 1 hour 59 minutes. SEAL training is much like that, too. Take one evolution at a time. Do what's in front of you, then the next thing, then the next. Just the thing that's in front of you. You keep that up long enough and you'll graduate BUD/S (Basic Underwater Demolition/SEAL) school.

So you need to do what's necessary. Your effort is a necessary thing. Your discipline is a necessary thing. Your intensity is a necessary thing. Nobody can sell you that. So nobody bothers talking about that because they can't package it up and give it to you.

Before all of these products made their way to the marketplace, people were fit. People were setting personal bests. They were amazing, their feats were astronomical, and nobody was handing them bags of protein powder to reach these goals.

In the 200,000 years that the human species has existed, the human body hasn't changed all that much. It's still made up of the same tissues, and it still takes competing against other humans to get you to points you didn't know existed. The athletes that I mentioned were leaders in their field because they had the will to train, the desire to win, and the discipline to follow through on all of it.

Will, desire, and discipline beat the shit out of everything.

If you have those three things, you can do anything.

THREE CORE PRINCIPLES

WILL

Will is the process by which people decide on and deliberately exert action/control to do something or to restrain their own impulses. When an actor knows that he's going to be shirtless for a portion of a movie and there's a lot of money riding on a picture, believe me he will be disciplined and will work hard toward making sure he looks his best. Actors don't want to be embarrassed. They don't want to let anybody down. And they care about their careers.

DESIRE

This is your motivation to do everything you can to achieve your goals. You've got to be 100 percent committed. I always say that you are better off with a 100 percent commitment and a half-ass plan than you are with a great plan and a half-ass commitment.

When I started training Chris Pratt, we were at a gym in Hollywood. Every day he showed up and gave it his all. The people in the gym would look at him like, *Who is this guy?* He gave every single rep his absolute best effort. He earned every drop of sweat. And look where his career went. He had the desire to transform himself.

DISCIPLINE

Be consistent. You've got to be disciplined enough to make sure you stick to the plan you have. That doesn't mean you won't have a setback. In fact, you will undoubtedly have a setback. But then you'll get back on track because your will and desire dictate that in order to get the results you want, you have to be disciplined enough to follow through. You have to be consistent. No one is doing this for you. This is all YOU. I said earlier that fitness starts with you. And it does.

―――――

If you have these three qualities, you will succeed. You can see it in people. They may get there at different times, but you just know it when someone is going to make it. They do so because they want to. There's not a damn thing anybody can do for you if you don't want to do it for yourself. And there's no amount of product, powder, or new workouts that will get you where you want to be.

I help my clients get there, but I don't do it for them. I can talk them out of a hole, but I can't make them lift a weight, force them to say no to a bowl of chips when they're at home, or to sleep enough for their bodies to recover.

That all comes from them.

In summary: Strength starts with you making a committed decision to get strong and the will, desire, and discipline to relentlessly pursue your goal: to get up every morning with your goal at the top of your list, to have reasons for doing this, not excuses.

Why be good when you could be great?

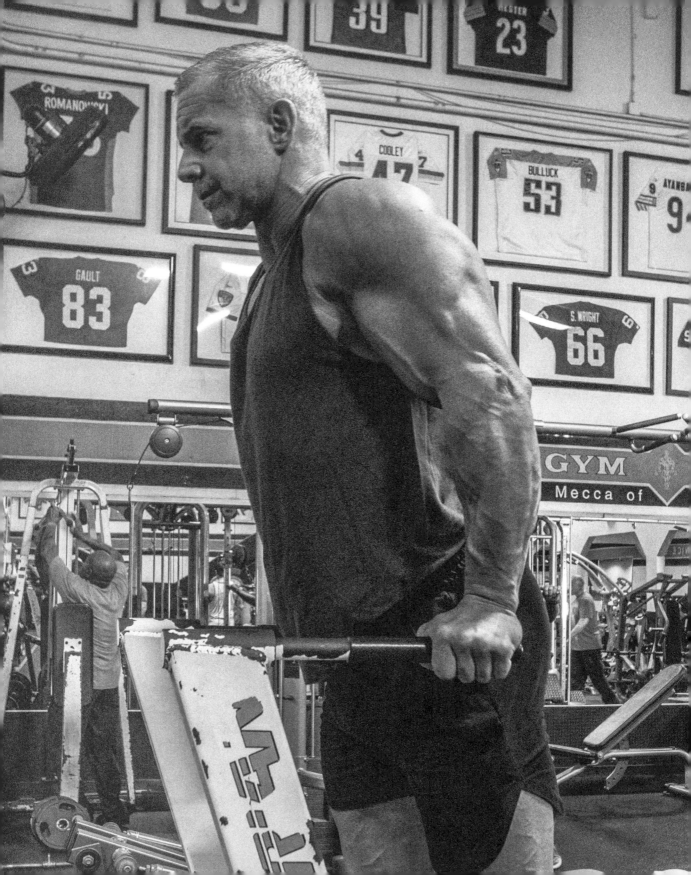

Why Are You Doing This?

Strength does not come from winning. Your struggles develop
your strengths. When you go through hardships and
decide not to surrender, that is strength.
—**Arnold Schwarzenegger**

GETTING FIT

The reality of getting ripped in twelve weeks is that it's possible but not probable for everyone. To pull this off, you've got to do a lot in a short amount of time, and you've got to nail it. For most people, this is not a realistic goal. It's a hope. So give yourself room to grow. You need to know this. I can't promise you instant success, even though my book's subtitle may make it sound like that. Can it be done? Sure, but not by everyone. This doesn't mean you won't get there over time. Some of you probably will pull this off, but most of you likely won't and shouldn't be discouraged by that in any way. So if in twelve weeks you are not Thor-ripped, that's okay. That's not how we measure progress (we'll get to that shortly). But if you listen to me and take my approach, I guarantee you that you will be heading in the right direction. When you are heading in the right direction, it builds your confidence; you'll find it easier to see where you are going. I am giving you the tools you need so that you can use all of them (exercise, proper nutrition, sleep, proper hydration, and being safe—because getting hurt sucks) toward reaching your goal.

There is no mystery to being fit. No one is born that way. But we're all born with the potential to be fit. Athletes don't get fit because they're athletic. They get fit because they capitalize on their potential and you have that opportunity as well. Actors and actresses don't get fit by snapping their fingers. They weren't born looking like that. And getting paid a lot of money doesn't get you fit. Neither does having some of the best plastic surgeons in the world on call or taking performance-enhancing drugs. They get fit because they really want to. They are all in. In the world of big-budget movies, they have to be fit, and they know that the way they look really sells a character. The celebrities that I work with take their training seriously because it impacts their careers.

When you first see Tobey Maguire get his powers in the original *Spider-Man,* you see the transformation his body undergoes, and he's in great shape. For the rest of the movie, that one shot of his body convinces the audience that he's Spider-Man. People buy into it. It's part of the role.

And sure, it's easier for my people than the general public. Most of my people have a specific goal in mind: the day he is shooting that scene with his shirt off or she is wearing that tightly molded superhero garb. There is no getting out of that. Your goal needs to be just as specific. This isn't impossible for you.

GUT CHECK

There're moments in SEAL training you could call the gut check. It's times in training when they ramp up the intensity to find out where guys breaking points are. Maybe you've heard of it. If you think you can't go on, then you've got to remind yourself how badly you want to do this. There might be times you want to quit. You won't, though, if you stay focused on your goals and accomplishing the task immediately in front of you. If my clients stray, I remind them what they are trying to do. You won't have me there with you, but that doesn't mean you can't check in with yourself now and then. To help keep you on the straight and narrow, add a reminder to your phone, write a note and tape it to your mirror, or check in with a buddy on a regular basis.

Give it a shot. It won't hurt you.

THE HIGHWAY TO SUCCESS

As far as I'm concerned, there are three possible ways to do things. The first approach is to get in your car and decide to drive on the autobahn, which means you are going to do everything I say from the exercise to the eating to the sleeping. You're all in. That's great. If you're that person, you will succeed. Then there are the folks that want to ride on the 405, which is good—you'll get your eating in as best you can, do the exercises, and get some sleep. Occasionally you may want to go out with your friends or have a beer. I wouldn't call this the best approach, but it's a start; in fact it may be where a lot of folks land. Finally, some folks will get in the car and drive along a back road, hitting every bump and pothole they can find, not giving a rat's ass what happens to their car. This is the wrong person to be. You will accomplish nothing.

You need to listen to me if you want this to work.

I need you to learn. Learning is so important.

Waiting for your turn to talk is not listening. Telling me about a diet your friend is doing is not listening.

If you hire me—and in buying this book you have hired me—let me do my job. I don't care what program you do, but do it all the way! Don't waffle around. A so-so plan executed with 100 percent conviction beats the hell out of an amazing plan carried out in a half-ass way. So imagine how well this is going to work if you have an amazing plan executed with 100 percent conviction.

THREE-LEGGED STOOL

I call this a three-legged stool. I don't refer to it as a principle, but if it helps you to think of it like that, you can. You've got to train amazing, eat amazing, and sleep amazing to look amazing. If any one of those legs falls off, obviously the stool isn't going to stand up.

I've been training Brad Pitt since 2003. He came to me when he was prepping for the role of Achilles in the movie *Troy*. He needed to pack size onto his legs. And let me tell you, it is *hard* to put size on your legs if you don't get it. That day I told him that "Discomfort is where the change takes place." Without saying a word, he grabbed a grease pen and wrote that phrase on the gym mirror. And I thought, *He's in, he's on board.* He was going to get this done. He understood how everything tied together. And he was going to trust me. On everything.

Every time you lift a weight, you've got to put a lot of effort into it. If you aren't, then what you are doing is too easy. It should be difficult. Every time you do cardio, the same thing is true. You're not on autopilot. You're putting a lot of effort into this. You've got to be safe and smart about it. Not reckless. Then you've got to take control of your diet. You've got to eat whole foods, real food all the time. You can't escape your physiology. You can burn only so many calories in a given amount of time. And you have to feed yourself. You have to feed yourself the nutrients to facilitate your life. Whether that's sitting at your desk and doing nothing or being a world-class athlete, you have to feed yourself the nutrients necessary for your lifestyle. If you want to get lean, you have to feed enough to the machine, but you've got to shortchange the extra calories. And your sleep has got to be good. You can't be staying up all night watching TV. You need to be on a schedule. Your body needs to rest as much as possible. Rest is how muscles repair themselves, how they grow stronger. It's also how you have the energy to beat them up again the next day.

THE WAY WE TALK TO OURSELVES

This is one of the most important points for you to grasp. The way we talk to ourselves affects so much of what we do and how we do it. Sometimes the only hurdles we have to get over are the ones we create for ourselves—in our minds. Getting rid of those impediments can be the difference between success and failure. And not just getting rid of them, but turning them into a way forward.

Oftentimes someone comes into my gym and says, "You know, Duff, I can't do this." Really? That's the first thing you say? You haven't even tried yet. Don't get in your own way. I guarantee you, you can do it. These are basic human movements. And yeah, most of the time the people that say this end up surprising themselves. Here's an experiment. Try adding the word *yet* to your sentence: I can't do this *yet*. That means you CAN do it. That means everything. Shift your perspective and your body will move with your mindset.

The SEALs and the Marines are big on making sure you give more than you think you can. Most of the time people are capable of doing more than they think they can. So in your mind you should never be thinking *can't* or *won't* or *don't*. Instead, you *will*. You will do more than you think you can do, and you're going to love how it makes you feel. You have to focus so that you don't get caught in the pitfalls of the things you are not comfortable with. Remember what Brad wrote on my wall: *Discomfort is where the change takes place.* Discomfort can mean so many things—straining under the effort of a weight, mentally pushing yourself when you *think* you have no more gas, or pushing thoughts from your head that stand in the way of your success.

Let's look at this another way. Have you ever watched Olympic downhill skiers when they are getting ready to do a run? They are at the top of that slope visualizing the run they are going to have. They know everything. The slope of the hill, the condition of the snow, the location of the turns—all of it. You never see them rehearsing failure in their head. It's the same for any pro athlete. A baseball player doesn't walk up to the plate visualizing whiffing against the pitcher. If he does, he's got a problem. No, he wants to get a base hit or crush a home run, so that's what he's thinking about.

When you come to me and say, "I can't" or "It's not happening," I'm not going to listen to that. Why would you come to me with that? You might say, "Well, that's how I feel." Okay then, I'll say, "Let's have a different conversation. Let's change the course of this dialogue."

There's a great saying in jiujitsu: "You don't lose, you either win or learn." So, for example, this could be the conversation in your head, and it's the type of thing I'll try to correct.

Negative: "What if something goes wrong?"

Positive: "What if everything goes right?"

Negative: "What if I can't do this?"

Positive: "What if you can?"

Do you get it now?

These changes to your thinking affect so much. What if the person you really want to look like is within your reach? A year from now you may look back on this—your struggle to change—and see the person you've become.

Wow. Get the fuck on board. Sign me up. This is the person I want to work with.

In the SEALs, people are elevated to a special status, giving them something to achieve, something to strive for. You're looking at this person, and you want to be like him or her. So in your case you are looking at someone with this amazing body and you want that body. Who do you think they are? They're you! That's it. They are you. They are you at this point in time, and they went down this road a while ago and incrementally worked their way toward this. This is who you are going to be in the future.

In SEAL training no one slaps a Budweiser in your hand when you get to the end. You work for it. There's a progression. You start out at a beginning level and the tasks get progressively harder. You're going to get good at swimming a mile before they have you swimming five miles. It works like that.

Nobody who became a SEAL or a Marine started out that way. That's day three hundred or year fifteen to get the kind of body you are looking for. SEALs or Marines didn't begin with that body. People assume that "I'm me and they're them." We're different.

No. You are not.

Those people are you. They're just heading along a different path, a path they started on a long time ago and one you are now embarking on.

Don't quit on yourself. You can get there.

When I was in my BUD/S training, I often stopped to realize that hundreds of men have done this before me—it's not like they came up with this yesterday and I'm the first guy doing it. Thousands did this before me. They were able to get through it, and they got fit to new levels.

I don't know what point B looks like for you, but you've got to head down that path and find out.

> ### EXPERT TIP
>
> You've got to cut yourself some slack, too. You're learning to behave in a different way. If fitness hasn't been a part of your life and you are trying to incorporate this line of being and you blow it, put that day behind you. There's no losing. There's learning. You know what you did wrong and you'll get it right the next time. Remember to talk to yourself as you would to your best friend. It's okay to be hard on yourself. But stay positive.

THE IMPORTANCE OF GOALS

I've said before how important it is to set specific goals, attainable ones. That's what keeps you going forward. That's how you avoid the pitfalls of thinking in the wrong way. If your goals are clear—if they are realistic and on point, and you are committed to them—you won't falter. When they're unclear or they're not realistic and they're weak, you struggle. If you believe in what you are doing and believe that you can go forward, you can and will. Then when you reach specific goals, you will set new ones. Until you get to exactly where YOU want to be. Not where someone like me wants you to be, not where your husband or wife wants you to be, but where you want to be.

YOU.

This journey is all about you.

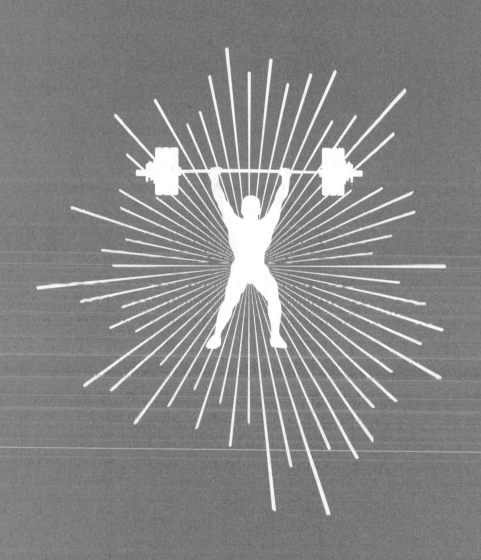

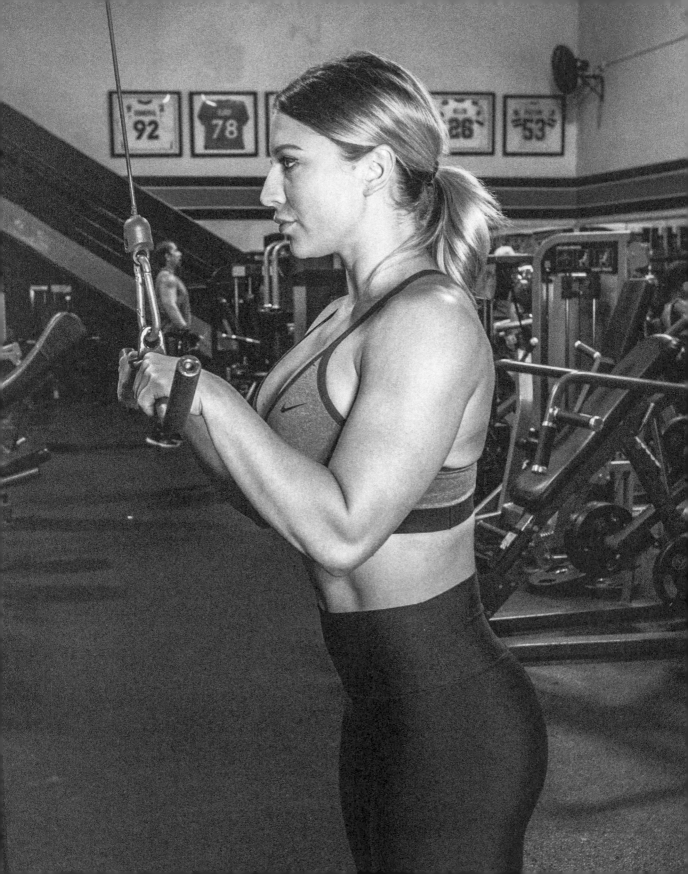

3

Measuring Progress

If you want be a lion, you must train with lions.
—Carlson Gracie, practitioner of Brazilian jiujitsu

WHAT IT TAKES

A lot of work goes into being a successful actor. You have to show up to an audition or a meeting, be told that you are ugly or that you are fat or too skinny or have a weird smile and you are not right for the part. There's a lot of rejection. A lot of people try to make it. Many of them go home. They don't make it. The people I work with got to where they are for a reason. They're not going to lose. They work hard. In a way, the attrition rate is worse than in the SEALs. My SEAL class started with around 120 guys and graduated 12 of them. There's a reason why there's only one Brad Pitt, Chris Hemsworth, or Scarlett Johansson. It's not an easy space to occupy. They're professionals to the end. They're also great role models for getting things done.

Look at what Chris Pratt did. This guy pretty much changed his life with fitness. He went from being a funny guy on a show to a mega-bankable movie star. He went from being unhealthy and overweight to looking like one of the fittest leading men in Hollywood. What I love about him is that he had 100 percent conviction in himself. He was getting this done when maybe other people didn't even think that he could. He worked so hard. He sweated it out at the gym. He got his mind right so he could eat right. He stopped going out and started taking care of himself. Because he cared. And if you ask him he will tell you, if he can do it, anybody can. He was 100 percent committed to driving on the autobahn. His transformation is inspirational. And he earned every bit of it. Guys like this are role models. Learn from them.

But again, you've got to be realistic about everything.

Will. Desire. Discipline. It all repeats.

EXPERT TIP: WHAT NOT TO DO

Once I was working with a forty-five-year-old woman. We talked and we exercised and she didn't express a clear goal of what she wanted. So I told her to come back the next day with a picture of the kind of look she wanted to get from our training. The next day she came in with a photo of what was probably a seventeen-year-old girl and said she wanted to look like that. Do you think that is realistic? Do you think she would ever get that look? No, she was setting herself up to fail. You have to take a look at your body type and your age, and figure out what it is you can do with the body that you have. It works only one way, and that's forward.

PROGRESS

So how I do measure someone's progress? Do I measure body fat? Not at all. I don't keep measuring devices around. There's no need. What good is it to know your body fat? If it's too high, you'll feel like it is not working. If it's low, it may not be an accurate representation of what's going on. You don't need to know your body fat, nor do you need to know what you weigh unless you are trying to lose a massive amount of weight. Even then I'm not so sure that that kind of knowledge is helpful because you will be gaining weight in the form of muscle. Progress is about how much you improve. That's the only measuring stick there is.

For example, if you can walk only a mile when you first start a program, but the next time you are able walk two miles, and by the third session you are able to do a light jog—that's terrific progress. If at first you can lift only a five-pound dumbbell and in a few weeks that five pounds is now twenty, you are doing an awesome job. When Brad Pitt started with me, he was doing bent-over rows with thirty pounds. By the time he was at the end of the program, he didn't even know that one day I had swapped out the weight he had been using and he was doing the same number of reps with ninety pounds. That's progress. If you use a rowing machine and in over half an hour you row 6,000 meters and then months later are able to row 7,000 meters in the same amount of time . . . Guess what? You've improved a lot.

I measure progress and success based on how much you improve. There's no greater measurement than that. And chances are, if you're improving, lots of positive changes are happening to your body. Your muscles are getting bigger. Your endurance is improving. Your body composition is changing.

Great! We're heading in the right direction.

EXPERT TIP

Say you have trouble staying motivated and you fall into a pit and it becomes a downward spiral. What do you do? Step forward. Do something. Put your gym stuff on. Put your shoes on. Sometimes it seems like there's a thing there. You get into a mindset where you are backing away. Don't back away. Lean in! Do it!

MASTERING MINDSET

I want you to be the best version of yourself. To do that, you've got to look at yourself and say *I can do this*. And if you can't and it's not for you, then stop. If you can't take this seriously, then you need to stop. Some people are going to be overweight. Exercise is not for them. But if you're going to be that way, then you need to be okay with yourself. Stop coming up with excuses. You want to eat that chocolate cake and complain about it—stop complaining. Just eat it and live. If that doughnut frustrates you, do something about it. Don't tell me or your best friend how it sucks; we all know it sucks. Go do something. Anything.

But if you want to be better, then you've got to get your mindset right.

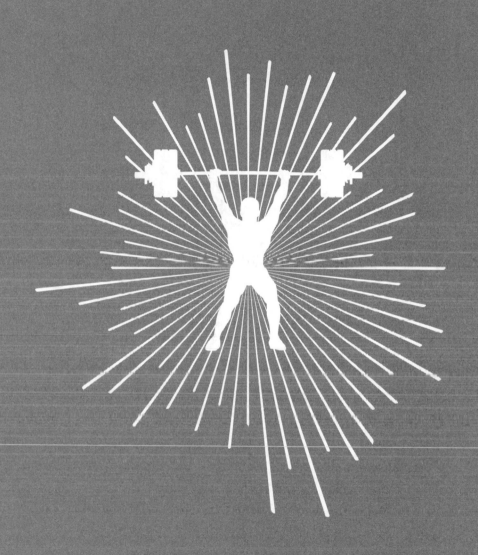

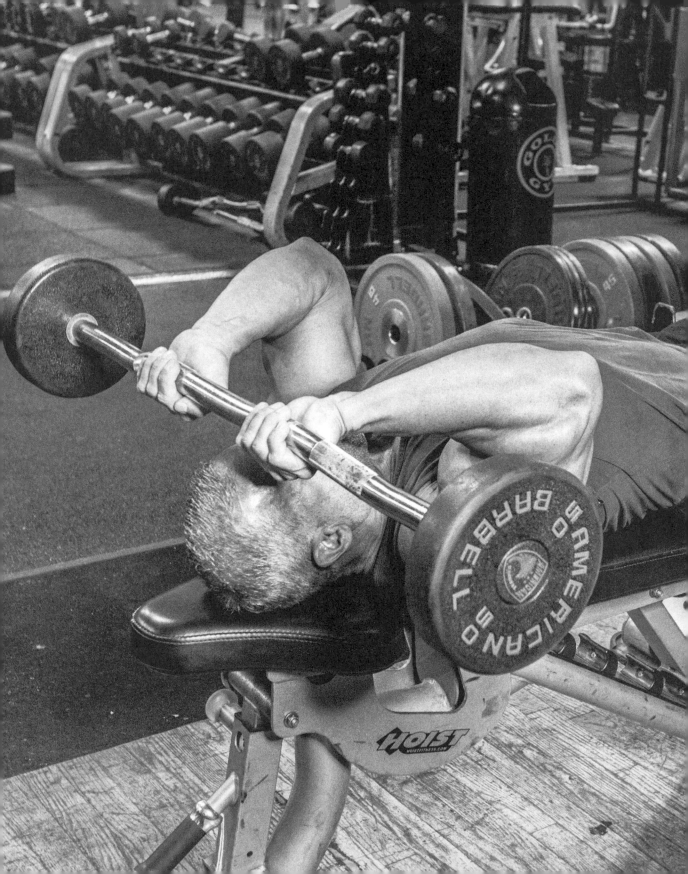

Introduction to the Exercises

You are the result of four billion years of evolutionary success. Fucking act like it.
—Anonymous

There is no one-size-fits-all approach to fitness. I have no idea what you look like. I don't know what your goals are. It's different for everybody. Maybe you want big shoulders, or maybe you just want to lose weight, or maybe you need to put on mass. Workouts and the types of workouts do different things for and to your body. The challenge of a fitness book is that it tries to get you as close to the trainer as possible, but it's not the same as having the trainer you want to work with. And most books are marketed with the idea that there is this one type of workout or a series of workouts or a style of workout that will get you where you need to go, and it's better than anything you've heard before. By now you know what my answer is to this. That's all great. But that's a marketing thing. It's not a fitness thing. Fitness hasn't changed. If you want big legs, you will squat and you will squat heavy weight. There's no way around that.

So I don't want you coming to these workouts I'm providing you with thinking that they are the answer and they are suddenly going to gift you with an amazing body. Sure, they are built on years of experience from reading, training, and exercising. They are proven and unquestionably will take you in the right direction if done right. At the end of the day, the most basic exercises work. There is no difference between biceps curls, alternating dumbbell curls, preacher curls, and cable curls. Rep and set schemes are endless options. The best results come from alternating between two basic rep patterns. One is lifting more weight for fewer reps, and the other is less weight for more reps. If you can do twenty reps, you should be adding weight. I'm going to give you the options for the exercises and some classic proven rep schemes. I've learned this stuff through trial and error and a lot of reading over the years. If your goal is greater size, these lower reps will serve you better for building strength; if you are already big and looking to lean out, these higher reps will help lean you out and improve your endurance. You should go back and forth. Go outside your comfort zone for the greatest change.

For example, I could draw a circle on the chalkboard and tell you to put in it the things you currently do for exercise, and you might write in there *doing CrossFit, running sprints, swimming,* and so forth. Now if I asked you what things you *don't* like to do, you might write down *body building* or *loaded carries,* putting them outside the circle. My response to your diagram would be that if you want to see tremendous change, *step out of your comfort zone.* If you've been doing one thing for years and not much has changed for you, it's time to try something new.

That said, everything works: body building, CrossFit, yoga, Tabata workouts. All of it. You can't go wrong. The area where people go wrong is in their heads. If you buy this book, the book isn't going to make you better. No piece of equipment you use will make you better, either. If you did any one of these workouts, they'd change your physique in some way for the better, especially if you are just rising up from the couch.

Statistically speaking, many people fail at this because it is so hard and because it is not an athletic thing and people think it is. It simply involves effort and mental discipline. These workouts may not be for you or they may be exactly for you. Everything works so long as you put in the effort.

Bench, squat, dead lift. If you did only those three exercises and were dialed in with everything on your nutrition, you would look fantastic.

You get this. You do. It's simple. All that is involved is basic exercises with some set patterns you can go with. As long as you move forward, you will bring about change for the better. Don't get hung up on what kind of running shoe you should or shouldn't buy. Just put on some shoes and go running.

Statistically speaking, you're not going to get in shape, otherwise there wouldn't be this epidemic of obesity. So the question is, are you going to step out of that norm? Are you going to buy the book and set it down? Are you going to use it as a coaster? Or are you going to get this done?

THE WORKOUTS

The workouts I'm giving you are the same ones I use with my clients. These are the same workouts that the A-list movie stars do. There's nothing different about them. Will they get you where you need to go? Of course. But it's going to be up to you to get there and to get out of them what you need. They're designed to give you a place to improve. As you get more experienced, you will need to build on them. If that means hiring a personal trainer, then do that. If that means talking to your friends who really know this stuff, then do that. Everything works. But what makes it the most effective is how you attack the workouts.

And go at your own pace. This isn't a race to see how fast you can dead-lift a truck. These are carefully structured workouts to bring out the best body you have in you. It's also not the only way to do things; it's just my way, and it's been quite effective for the clients I train.

I don't want you getting hurt. I want you exercising smart. When you get hurt, then you can't exercise and that's not smart. It's also not good for your body.

So you need to go slow and steady and focus on every lift that you do.

WARMING UP

At the start of every workout, you should warm up. This is really important, and even more essential for people as they get older. You need to loosen up your muscles. You need to get your blood flowing and your heart rate up. All of this is proven to help prevent injury and primes your body for strenuous activity. *But what about stretching?* you might ask. I would tell you that stretching is not as important as warming up and is usually just a distraction for people. I don't want you to create a hurdle. People get too wrapped up in that stuff. *But you have to stretch—everyone says so.* Wrong. In fact, it's not even totally necessary. How you warm up is up to you. And again, there is no one way to do it. Whatever works for you. Go for a jog, do jumping jacks, use a rowing machine. Your primary goal is to make sure that you have blood flowing to the muscles and that your heart rate is elevated enough so that you can start exercising with a lot of effort.

ECCENTRIC VS. ISOMETRIC VS. CONCENTRIC

You've probably heard these terms before. They're important to understand. A concentric contraction causes the muscles to shorten, thereby generating force. For example, let's say you are curling a weight. This is when you are exploding upward with the weight. Eccentric contractions cause muscles to elongate in response to a greater opposing force. So if you are curling a weight, on the lowering portion of the exercise you are slowly bringing it back down to stress the muscles. Isometric contractions generate force without changing the length of the muscles. If we again use the example of curling the weight, here you are using a weight that is too heavy for you and you can hold it in place but you can't lift it up.

HOW YOU LIFT THE WEIGHT IS JUST AS IMPORTANT AS THE WEIGHT YOU ARE LIFTING

So to build the most muscle, to get the most bang for your buck, lifting would work like this. Let's say you can curl a 40-pound dumbbell, but that's your limit. So you may not be able to curl this 45-pound dumbbell but you can hold it isometrically mid-curl. And you can't hold a 50-pound dumbbell, but you are capable of lowering it in a controlled eccentric motion. In a perfect world, I'd have you curl a 40-pound dumbbell up explosively (concentric)—you can handle that weight versus the 45-pound dumbbell—and then on the way down I'd swap it out for a 50-pound dumbbell for the eccentric portion of the exercises. We'd do this with every rep. So it'd be up with 40 pounds, followed by an isometric hold with 45 pounds, and then down with 50 pounds each time. Since we don't have that option, what we'll do is have you explode up concentrically with the 40-pound dumbbell, squeeze for a beat (isometric), then slowly lower the weight on the eccentric portion of every rep, trying to mimic what would happen if the dumbbell had actually changed weight. This is the most effective way to stimulate growth, to get the most out of every single rep.

What I teach my clients is that every rep matters. It isn't about doing dozens of sets and endless varieties of exercises. It's about using the most effort during every single rep that you take no matter what exercise you are doing. Don't be so concerned about how much weight you are lifting. Be more concerned about how you are lifting that weight. Are you using it to your fullest advantage? This method of lifting builds the most muscle. It's the fastest method and it challenges you.

So when you approach the workout that I've written for this book or any of the other workouts included in this book, the only way you should be lifting is this way. It can be applied to everything: sit-ups, crunches, bench presses, etc. I want to really hammer this home. You may look at one of these workouts and think, *Boy, that looks easy.* Well, if you are doing it right, if you are giving it maximal effort and performing lifts explosively on the way up and eccentrically on the way down, it shouldn't be easy. Sweat should be dripping off your body when you do these workouts. When I'm at a gym with a client who is getting ready for a role, people often stare at them, and they're not staring at them because of who they are. They are staring at them because they can't get over how much my clients are sweating and how hard they are working to try to transform their body. This is the mindset you need to have when you exercise.

PRACTICE GOOD FORM

You hear that a lot, but what does it mean? It's partly a disclaimer in case you hurt yourself and sue. Obviously if someone gets hurt, he or she wasn't practicing good form so my club or program is off the hook.

Good form basically means this: Don't throw the weight around. If you can't actually curl the 100-pound easy curl bar, don't pick it up and start swinging it around as if you can. Use the least amount of weight to get the job done.

Keeping good form in mind, milk every ounce of growth out of every rep, which means exploding (but in total control) for more muscle fiber recruitment on the concentric portion of the exercise, an isometric squeeze at the top of the rep, and a slower eccentric portion of the rep.

BREATHING

When you are lifting weights you should always be breathing out on exertion. For example, if you are performing the bench press, you are inhaling as you lower the weight to your chest and breathing out as you explosively push it up.

BASIC EXERCISES TO KNOW

In the next section are the exercises you need to know. For anything you have questions about, I highly recommend you do some research online or talk to a friend or trainer who knows what he or she is doing. There are a ton of resources out there. You don't want to guess your way through something. And for those of you who know this stuff, although refreshers are always a good idea, you can skip ahead to the chapter that works for you.

If you're starting from a place of no prior training or you have little upper body mass, then you will need the bench presses to be a part of your program, but if you have achieved a reasonable amount of size in your chest, you can maintain a reasonable amount of size with push-ups and some dumbbell work. I've had many a conversation with clients through the years on what a good male physique looks like, and we always end up agreeing that a large chest looks like a guy that goes to the gym a lot, whereas a smaller ripped-up chest with a wide back, larger shoulders, and thick arms looks more natural, as if it came about through work instead of through attendance at a gym.

CHEST AND TRICEPS EXERCISES

BENCH PRESS

There are different ways to bench press. You set up differently if you are a powerlifter, for example. If that's your thing, great. I'm not going to cover that here. I want to make sure you have an understanding of the fundamentals. For your bench press, lie down on the bench so that your head is just slightly ahead of the bar. You take your grip with your hands approximately in line with your shoulders. Some people like to grip it wide, others close. These variations are okay. Just understand the farther away your arms get from your body, the more strain you put on your shoulders. I like to be safe, so I suggest shoulder width. Wrap your hands around the bar, squeeze it, and take it out of the rack. Once it is over you, you want to make sure your glutes are on the bench, your shoulder blades are pulled toward each other, and your traps are digging into the bench. Your head is neutral. It shouldn't ever move unless you like having neck problems. Take a breath, hold it, then as you exhale, lower the bar steadily. Your elbows should brush your sides as you bring the bar toward your body. Do not ever let your butt leave the bench. This is important for the safety of your back and spine. You will see people doing this at the gym. It's a terrible idea—idiotic, in fact. Feel the stretch then push the bar back up while breathing out. This exercise can also be performed with dumbbells if that's all you have access to.

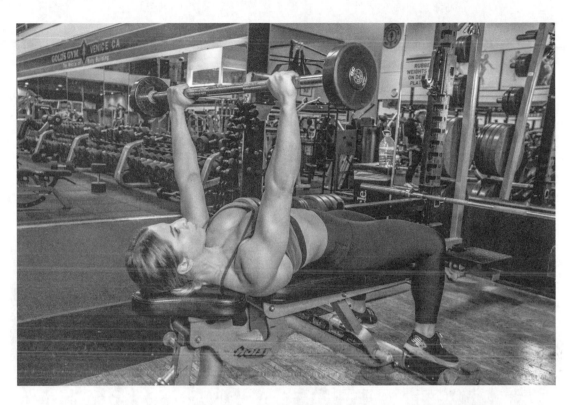

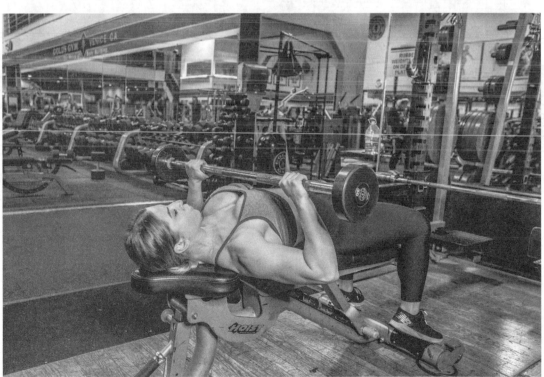

LYING TRICEPS EXTENSIONS

Lie on your back on a weight bench, feet flat on the floor. Using dumbbells or an EZ curl bar, hold the weight above your shoulders. Bend your arms at the elbows, bringing the weight down above the head, stretching the triceps. Then raise the dumbbells or EZ curl bar back up. Do not let your elbows flare out.

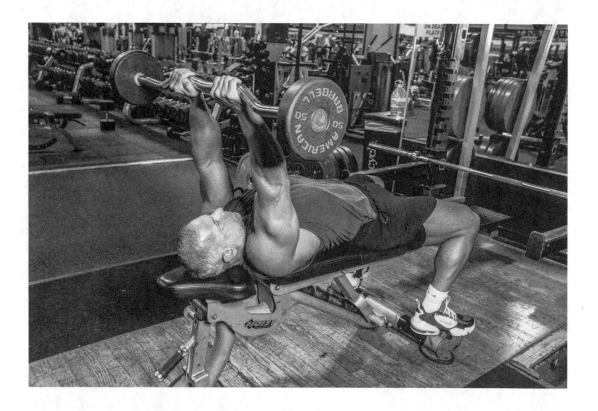

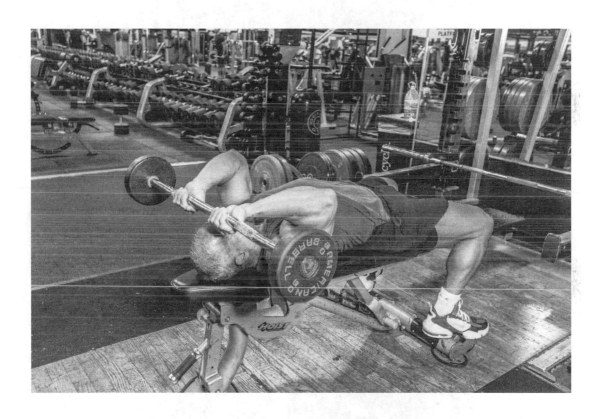

CABLE TRICEPS PUSH-DOWN

Stand in front of a bar or rope on a cable station. With your elbows bent, arms somewhat close together, and palms down, grasp the bar or rope and push the weight down using your triceps. When your arms are fully extended, hold for a few seconds, and then slowly raise your hands and repeat.

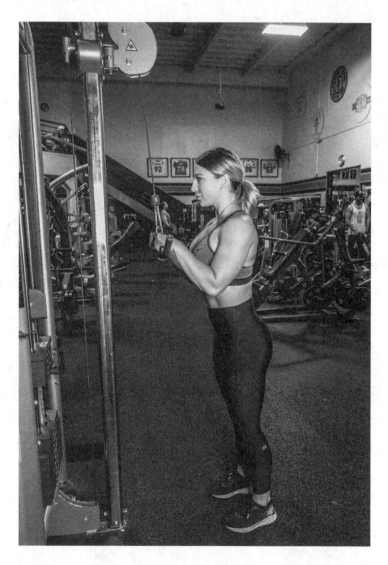

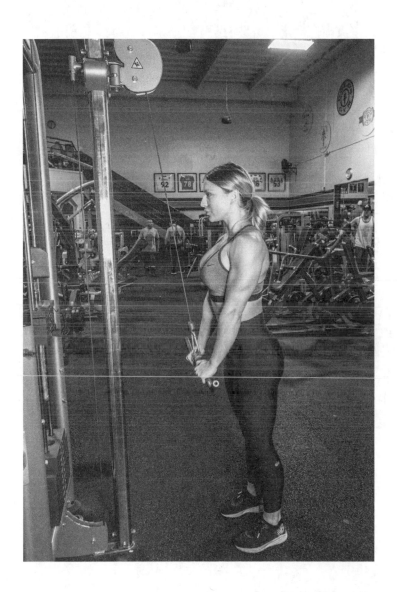

VARIATION
(Not Pictured)
**REVERSE
SINGLE-ARM
TRICEPS
PUSH-DOWN**

Grab the
D handle with
your palm
facing up and
slowly lower it
until it is at your
side. Then raise
and repeat.

DIP

You need to use a dip bar. This is one of the most efficient ways to build triceps, shoulders, and chest. You hold on to the dip bar and lower yourself to about where your elbows are halfway bent. You don't want to go too deep and you also don't want to shortchange yourself by not going down far enough. That's one rep. You can add weight to these using a dip belt if you are proficient at them.

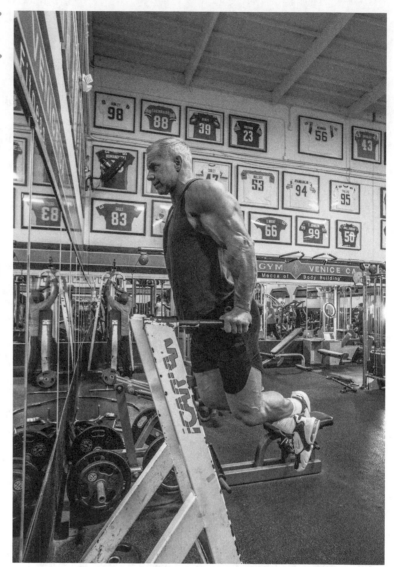

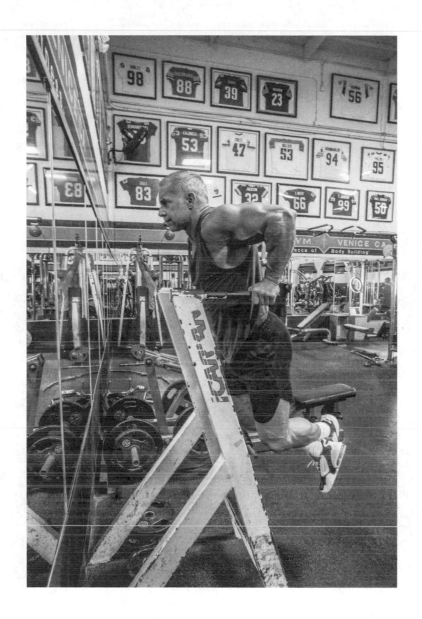

DUMBBELL FLYES

Lie back on a bench holding the dumbbells over your shoulders. Keeping a slight bend in your elbows, lower your arms out in a wide arc until you feel a stretch on your chest. Squeeze your chest muscles as you return your arms to the starting position, then repeat. Be sure to keep your elbows bent and don't lower your arms below the bench.

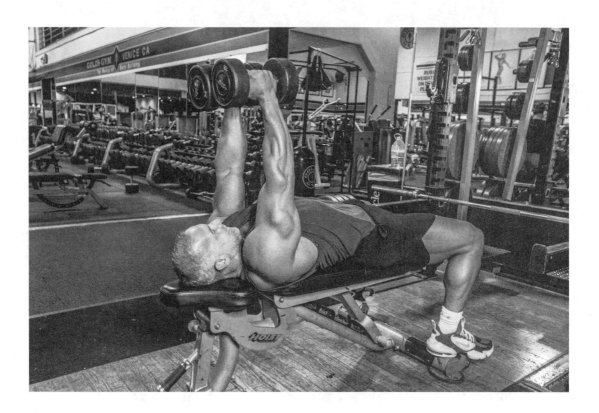

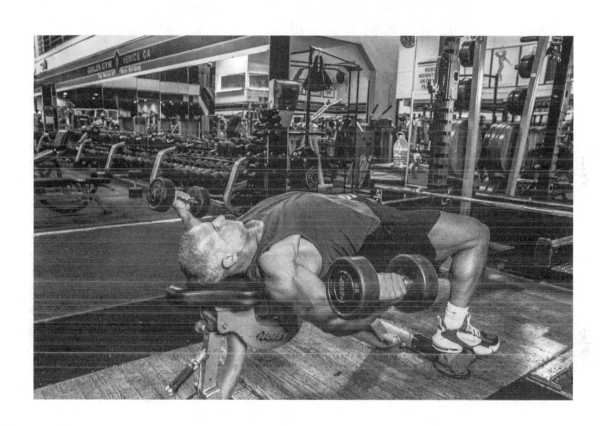

PUSH-UP

Place your hands directly below your shoulders and lower yourself to the ground so that your chest touches. Then push yourself back up.

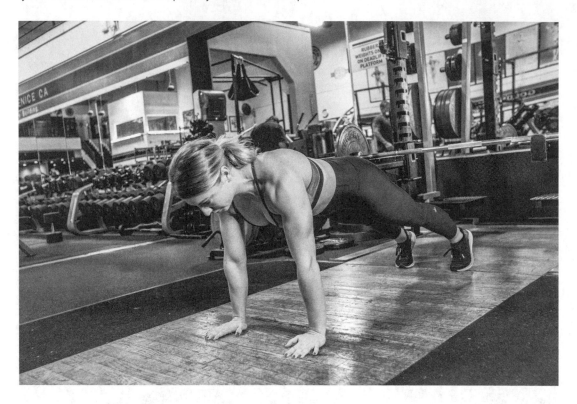

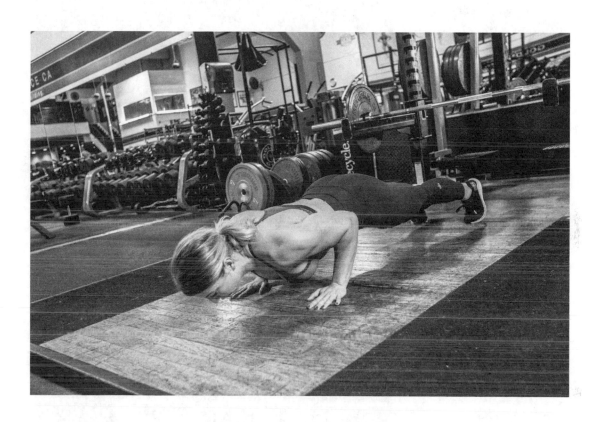

VARIATION (Not Pictured) DIVE BOMBER PUSH-UPS

Get into a push-up position and then push your hips up as high as possible. You should resemble an inverted V. Lower your hips, keeping your legs straight, but allow your arms to bend as you push forward so that your chest nearly grazes the floor. Press back through your hands to full arm extension and then reverse the sequence. This counts as one rep.

DUMBBELL KICKBACK

Lean forward, keeping your back straight with a slight bend in the knees, or rest one hand on a bench. Your torso should be almost parallel to the floor. Holding the weight in your hand extend your arm back, tightening the triceps, pause, and then slowly return the arm to the starting position. Repeat on the other side.

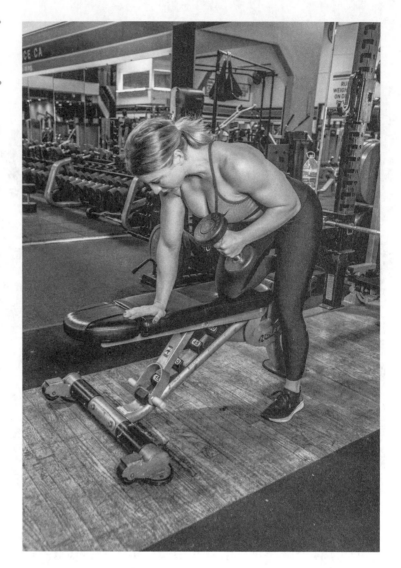

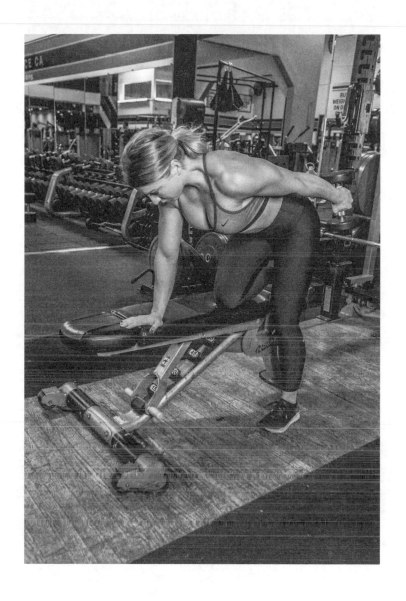

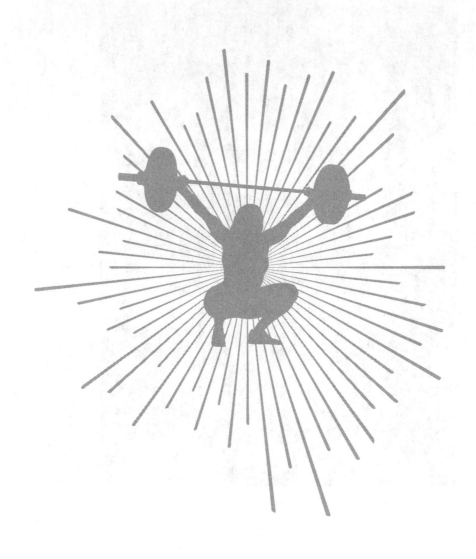

SHOULDER EXERCISES

MILITARY PRESS

Set the bar so that it is just above head height. Go under the bar and take it out of the rack. The bar should be resting on or near your clavicle, slightly tucked under your head. Feet should be about shoulder width. Now as you begin the lift, you want to push the bar up toward your chin, making sure you don't hit yourself, and then extend the bar past your face and over your head with a good stretch. You do not want to push it straight up. It should be going up and back over your head. You want that stretch to keep your shoulders pliable. You can also perform this exercise with dumbbells. And it is perfectly fine to perform the lift in a split stance, which can reduce the hyperextension of the spine and pelvis.

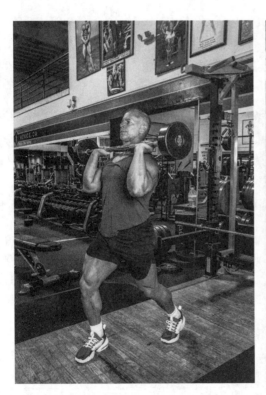 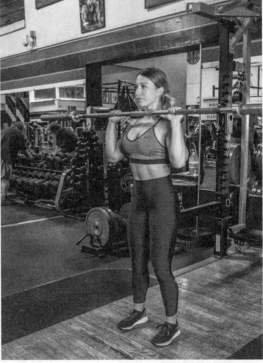

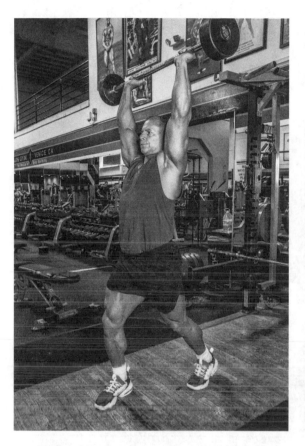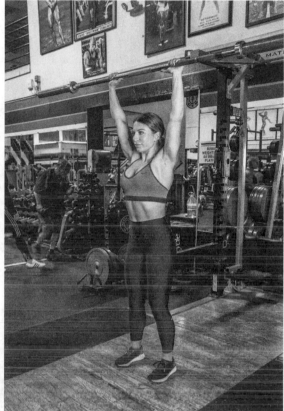

VARIATION (Not Pictured) PUSH PRESS

This is similar to the military press. Holding the bar just above the collarbone, slightly flex the hips and knees and explosively push upward by straightening the knees. You want full extension. Lower the bar back down and repeat.

ARNOLD PRESS

This is a variation on the military press. Hold the dumbbells up in front of you around shoulder level, palms turned toward you. Raise the dumbbells to the full extension of your arms, rotating the palms so they are facing forward. Now slowly lower your arms, turning the palms toward you, and repeat.

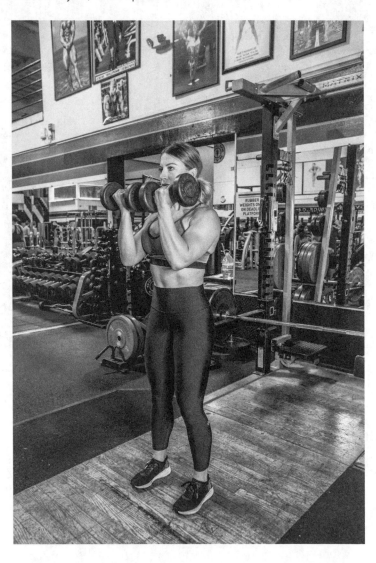

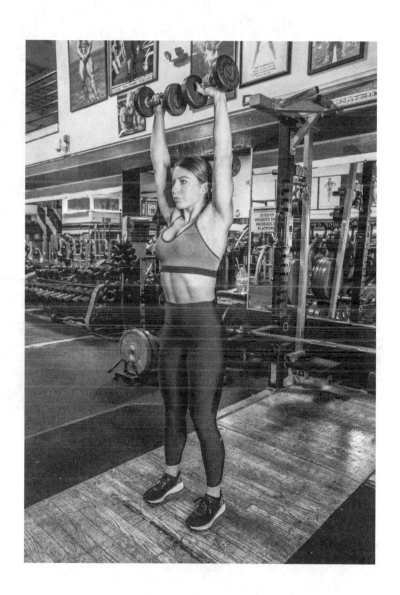

REAR DELT RAISES

Holding a dumbbell in either hand, bend forward at a 45-degree angle, keeping your back straight. Raise the dumbbells out to either side, taking care not to go above shoulder height. Squeeze your delts and then lower and repeat.

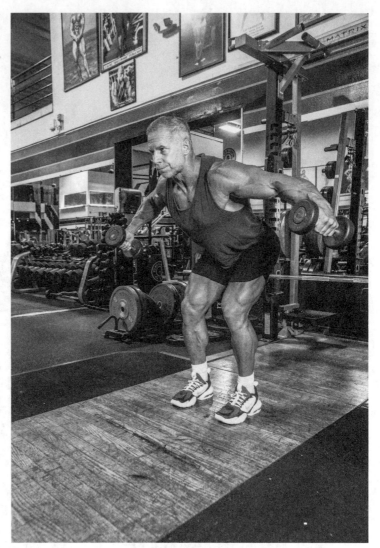

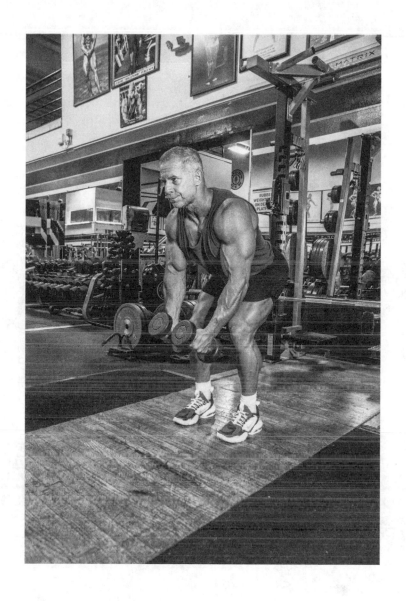

LATERAL DUMBBELL RAISE

Standing upright, grasp a dumbbell in either hand, with palms facing inward. Keeping your elbows slightly bent, raise your arms out to the sides until they're at shoulder level, pause, and then lower the weights back to the starting position.

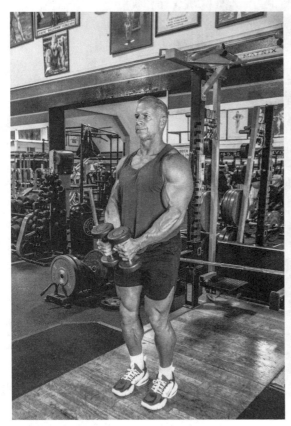 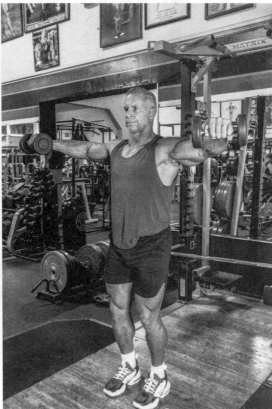

FRONT DUMBBELL RAISE

Stand with knees slightly bent, arms straight down in front of you, holding a dumbbell in either hand. Palms should be turned toward your body. Keeping your arms straight, raise both of them up slowly to shoulder height, hold for a second, then lower them back down.

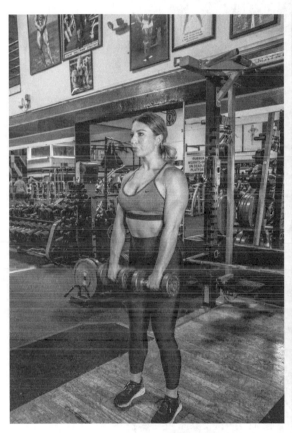
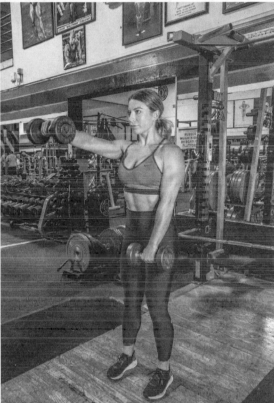

UPRIGHT ROW

Grasp a barbell with an overhand grip that is slightly less than shoulder width. You can also use a pair of dumbbells for this exercise. Bending your elbows, lift the bar up until it nearly touches your chin. Pause for a second at the top before lowering back down.

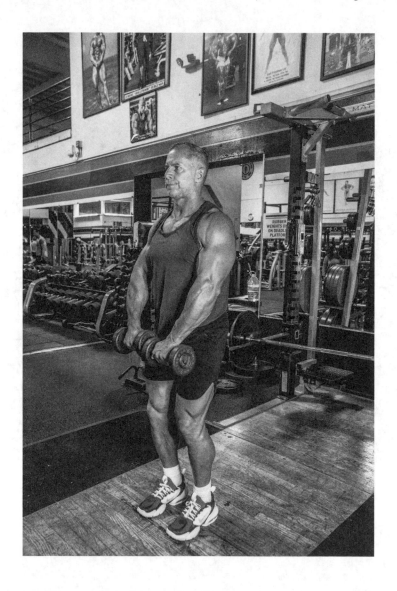

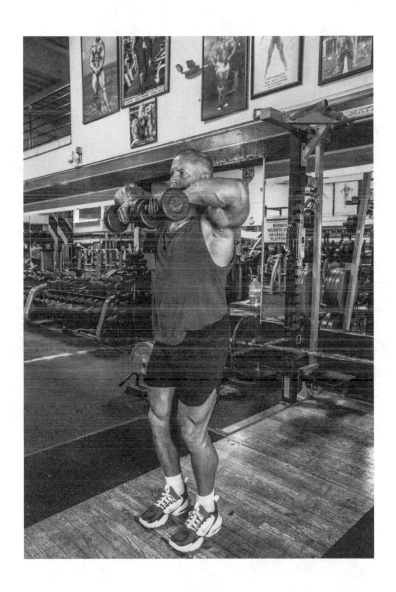

BRAD PITT—June 17, 2003

LEG DAY
Superset:
Leg extensions 90 lb × 15, × 15, × 15, × 15

Push-ups × 15, × 12, × 12, × 12

Sit-ups × 15, × 15, ×15, × 15

Squats 50 lb × 20, 135 lb × 15, 165 lb × 15, 185 lb × 15,
205 lb × 12, 225 lb × 10, 245 lb × 8

Leg press 90 lb × 20, 140 lb × 20, 180 × 20, 180 × 20
Leg curl 60 lb × 15, 70 lb × 12, 70 lb × 12, 70 lb × 10,
70 lb × 10

Standing calf raises 100 lb × 20, 110 lb × 20, 120 lb × 18,
130 lb × 17

LEG EXERCISES

BACK SQUAT

The bar should rest in the rack about shoulder height. You come up under it and settle it onto your back, just under the neck, on the shelf of your shoulders. Don't take too many steps back—it wastes energy. Grip the bar hard and keep your elbows in tight. Set your feet slightly past shoulder width, but not too wide; in the squat you want to sit back and open up your hips. Your eyes remain straight ahead and your neck neutral. When you begin your descent, push your knees out to the sides and your glutes back. You're going to come down to where your thighs are parallel with the ground, but it's even better if you can get below parallel, to the point where your hamstrings touch the back of your calves. This can also be done with dumbbells at your side or holding one dumbbell in front of you or simply without weights (air squats).

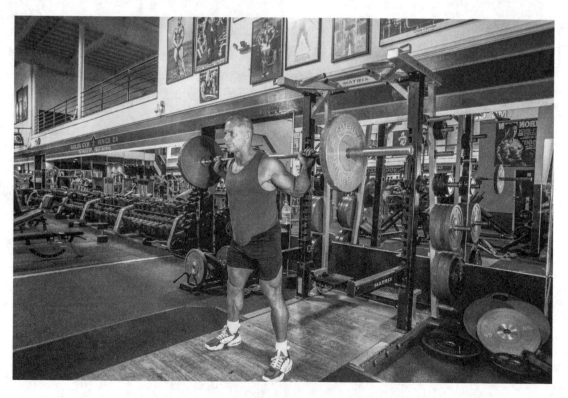

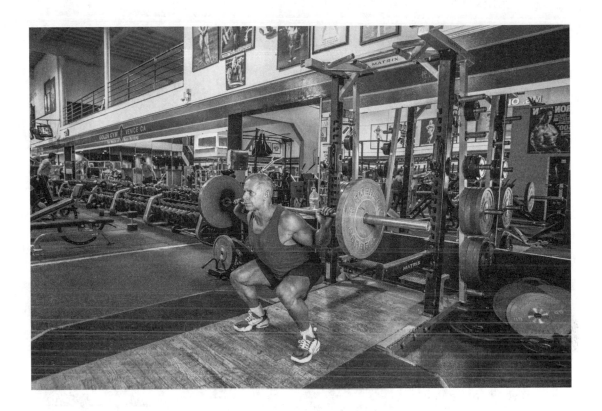

VARIATION (Not Pictured) BREATHING SQUATS/SETS OF 20

After you become familiar with squats, one highly effective form of squatting is a breathing squat, in which you do lots of reps, like sets of 20, and you push through the pain to accelerate your metabolism. This is an old body builder technique and important to know. Step back, take a deep breath, and begin. Squat all the way down, at least to where your thighs are parallel to the ground. Come back up, take a few deep breaths, and squat again. As you get further into the set, breathing may become an issue. Take as many deep breaths as necessary between reps. You must keep complete focus throughout the entire set.

FRONT SQUATS

Start with the bar secure in the squat rack, level with the middle of your chest. Hold the bar with hands just wider than shoulder width apart. Step in close to the bar and lower into a quarter squat so the bar is level and touching the top of your chest and the front of your shoulders. Without letting go of the bar, bring your elbows forward and up as high as you can manage. Focus on keeping your elbows as high as possible throughout the squat; this will keep your body upright and the bar secure in the crook of your hands and resting against your chest and shoulders. Drive up

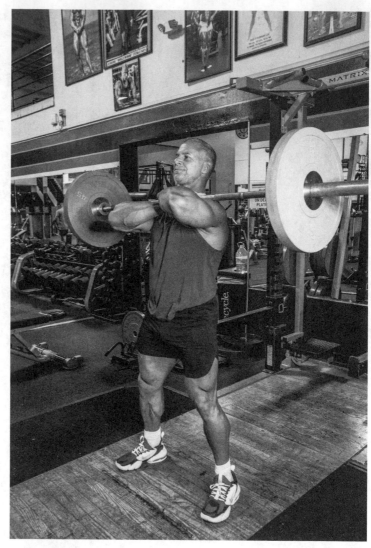

to take the bar out of the rack. Position your feet shoulder width apart, with your toes slightly turned out. Brace yourself, take a deep breath in to fill your chest and keep your torso strong, then bend your knees to lower into a squat. Keep your knees wide apart, with heels down. Lower until your thighs are at least parallel to the floor, then drive back up to stand.

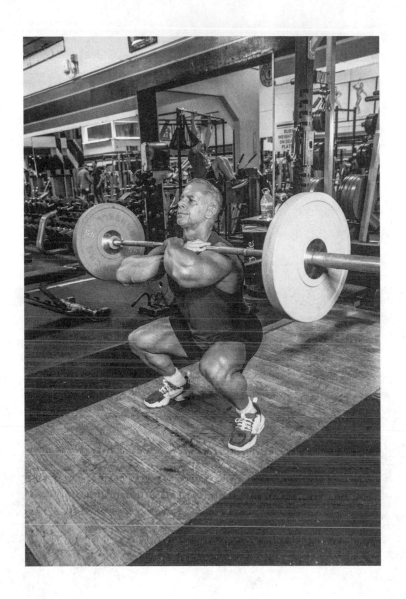

HACK SQUAT

With a barbell placed behind you, stand up straight, with your feet at shoulder width. You're going to squat down and reach behind you to grab the bar with a shoulder-width grip and your palms facing behind you. Stand up holding the bar, and then squat back down, taking the bar to the floor and then back up again while keeping your head and eyes up and back straight. Inhale as you slowly go down. Pressing mainly with the heel of the foot and squeezing the thighs, stand back up as you breathe out. You can also use a machine. You set up and squat down and then push yourself back up.

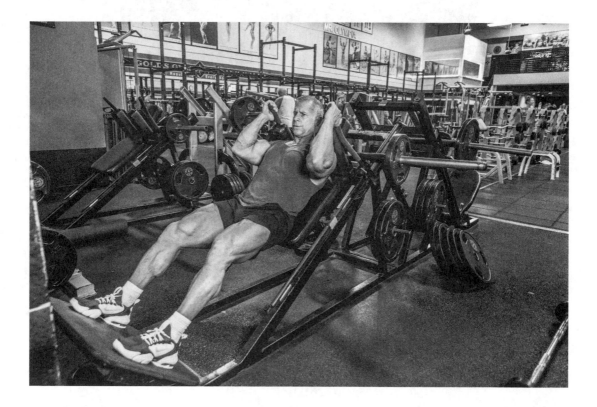

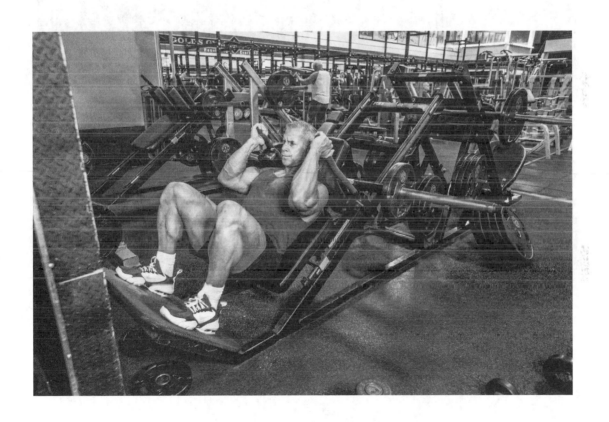

LEG PRESS

Using a leg press machine, set your desired weight. Position your feet at approximately shoulder width and press the weight up. Then slowly bend the knees and return to the starting position. Repeat to your desired reps.

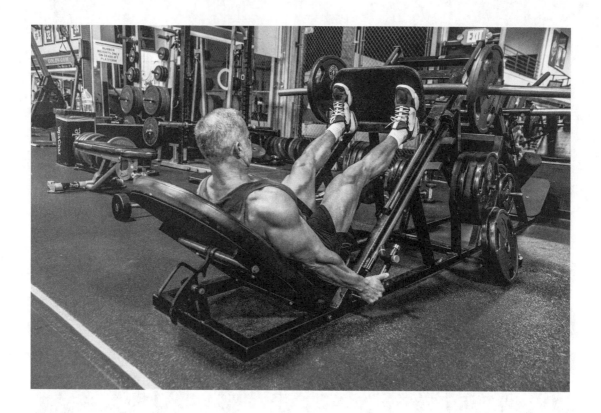

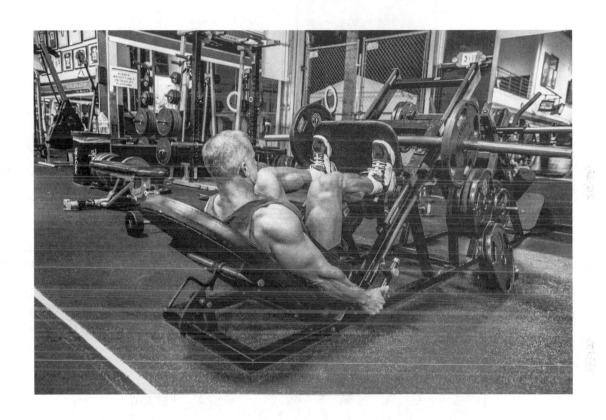

LEG EXTENSION

You'll need a leg extension machine. Once you are in position with the proper weight set, use your quads to straighten your legs as you exhale. Slowly bend your knees and lower the weight back to the starting position.

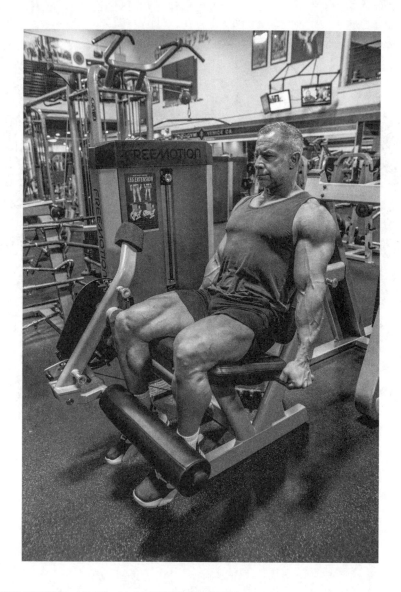

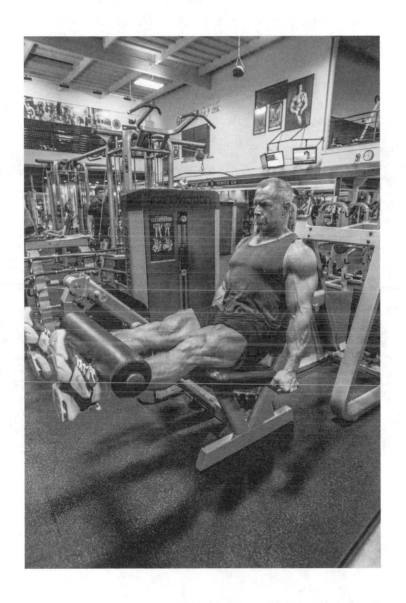

LEG CURLS

Find a leg curl machine, get in it, and curl the weight up to the back of your hamstrings. Then slowly straighten your legs and lower the weight to the starting position. If you don't have access to a leg curl machine, you can substitute a dumbbell. Lie facedown on a bench and clamp the weight between your ankles. Proceed as with a machine.

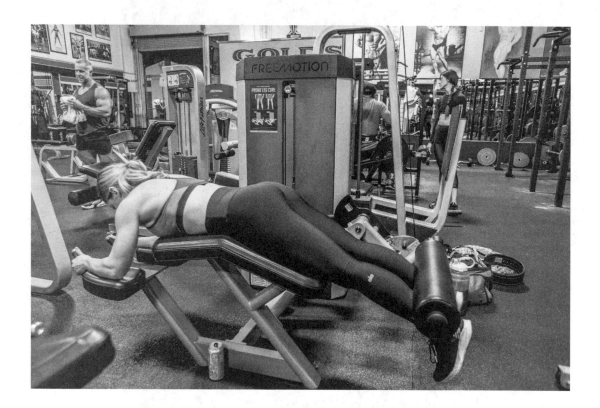

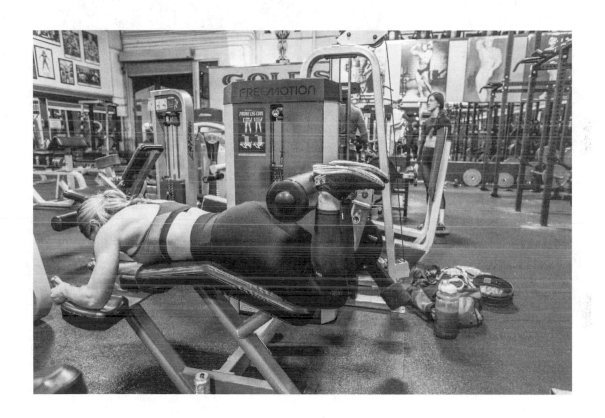

CALF RAISES

Your feet should be parallel to each other, not turned in or out. Raise yourself up as high as possible by flexing your calf, hold for a moment, and then go back down slowly and stretch the calf out. If you don't have a machine, grab some dumbbells. Position yourself on the edge of a stair or on the floor and just raise yourself up on your toes and then lower yourself down.

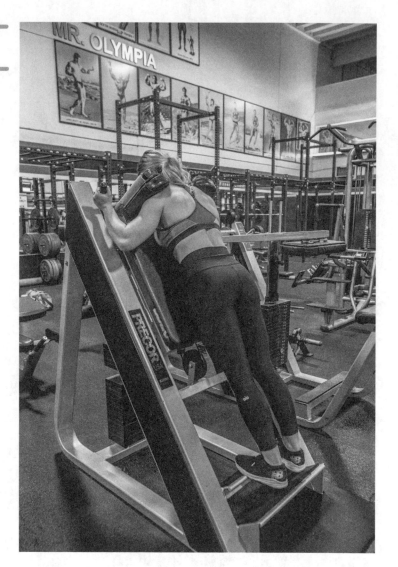

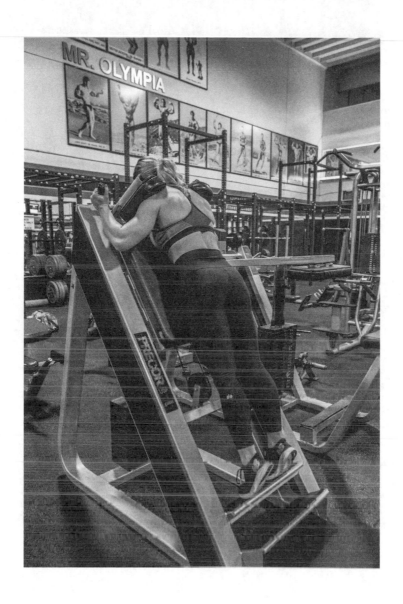

CHRIS HEMSWORTH — March 14, 2011

BACK & BICEPS

Pulldowns Hammer Strength 90 lb × 20, 140 lb × 15, 180 lb × 15, 230 lb × 12, 270 lb × 10, 300 lb × 8

Dumbbell rows 65 lb × 15, 70 lb × 15, 75 lb × 12, 80 lb × 10, 85 lb × 10, 90 lb × 10

Dumbbell curls 30 lb × 15, 35 lb × 15, 40 lb × 15, 45 lb × 12, 50 lb × 10, 45 lb × 6, 40 lb × 6, 35 lb × 11, 30 lb × 15

Hyperextensions × 15, × 15, × 15

Abs (sit-ups × 25, crunches × 25, seated twist with 10 lb ball × 25) × 4 rounds

BACK AND
BICEPS EXERCISES

DEAD LIFT

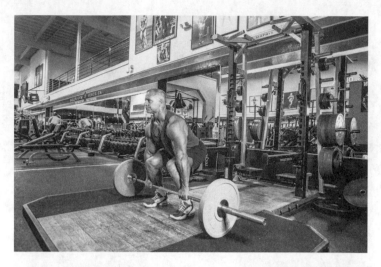

You want to place your feet just inside shoulder width, although some people like to have them at shoulder width. Experiment with what works best for you. Sometimes checking where your feet are when you jump is a good place to work from. Your shins should be just a touch away from the bar, maybe about an inch. You then bend over and grasp the bar with both hands. There are two grips. One is with both palms facing forward, which keeps the muscles balanced and is good for working on grip, but when you go heavy, you usually need to have a mixed grip,

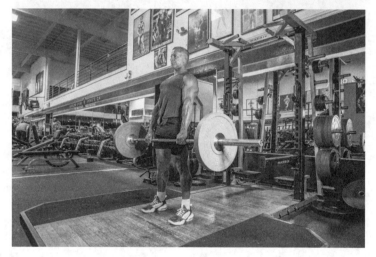

where one hand is under the bar and one is over. Usually your dominant hand is the one that is over. You then bend slightly at the knees, sit your hips back, and lift the bar. You need to keep your chest up and your back neutral as you lift. Then you lock it out so that you are nearly vertical. Afterward, lower the bar steadily to the ground. Don't drop or slam the weight. If you do that, you are only cheating yourself. The process of lowering the bar back down builds strength as well.

SUMO DEAD LIFT

Your feet should be set very wide. Arms should be below the shoulders, inside the legs. Grasp the bar with palms away from you or with palms toward you, or with a mixed grip (one palm away, one palm toward you). Take a breath and then bend your knees and lower your hips, chest up and face forward. Drive through the floor, and extend through the hips and knees. As the bar passes through the knees, lean back and drive the hips into the bar, pulling your shoulder blades together. Return the weight to the ground in a controlled fashion.

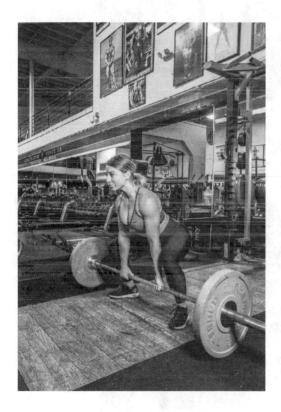 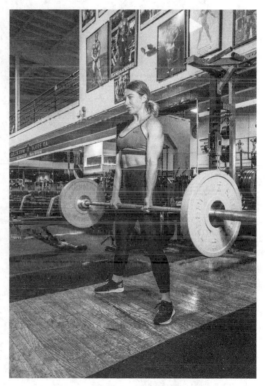

T-BAR ROWS

Bend over the bar until your torso is at a 45-degree angle to the floor. Attach a double D handle and use it to pull the weight up to your abdomen. Hold for a moment and then lower the bar.

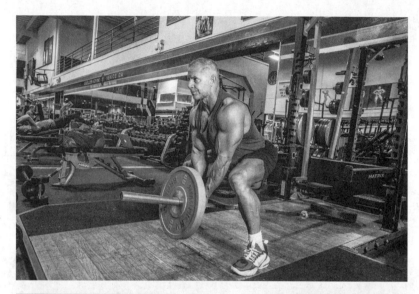

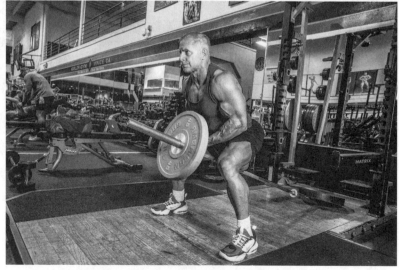

CABLE ROWS

Sit at a cable row station. Using a D handle and keeping a neutral back, pull the weight toward you until your arms just touch your abdominals. Squeeze your back and then slowly return the D handles to the starting position.

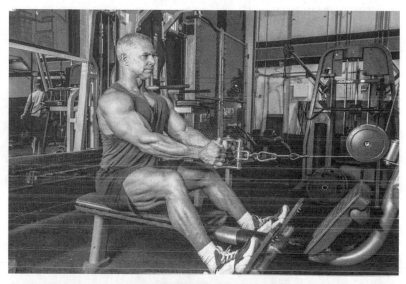

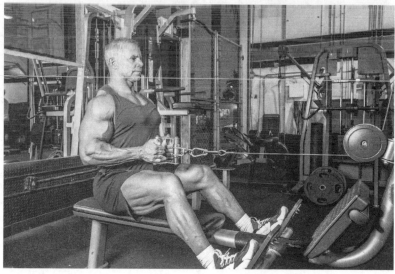

BENT-OVER BARBELL ROW

Using a pronated grip on the barbell, bend forward slightly at the waist, keeping knees slightly bent and your back neutral. Pull the weight up to just below your ribs, squeeze the back, and lower the barbell back down.

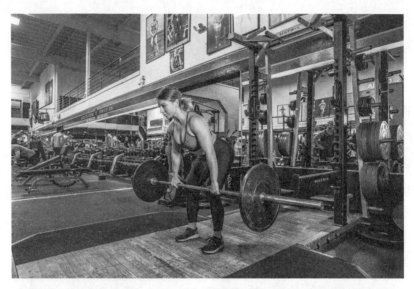

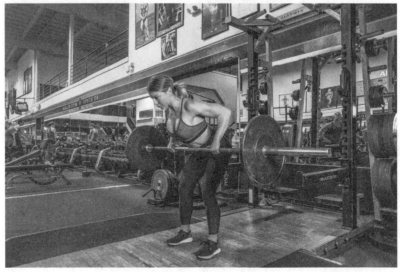

DUMBBELL ROW

With one hand on a bench for support, hold a dumbbell in the other hand and bend forward slightly. Pull the dumbbell up toward your rib cage and then lower it back down. Repeat on the other side.

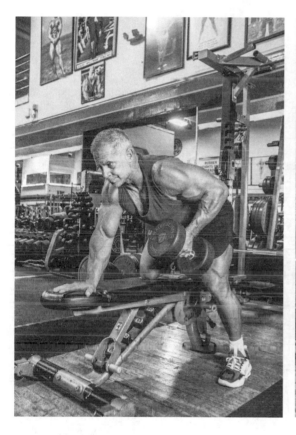
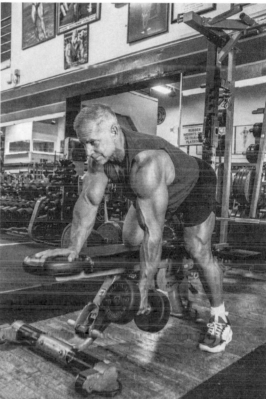

BARBELL CURL

Start holding a barbell at a shoulder-width grip. The palms of your hands should be facing forward and the elbows should be close to the torso. Keeping your arms stationary, curl the weight forward and upward while contracting the biceps. Lower the weight back down slowly and repeat.

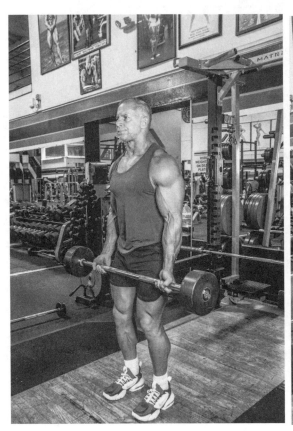 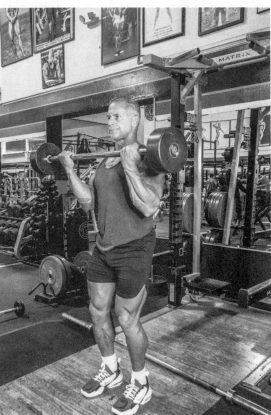

DUMBBELL CURLS

This exercise can be done standing or seated on a weight bench. Start with weights in your hands, palms turned toward your side. Your elbows should be close to your torso. Keeping your arms stationary, curl the weight forward and upward while contracting the biceps. The palm of the hand should rotate toward the body. Lower the weight back down slowly and repeat.

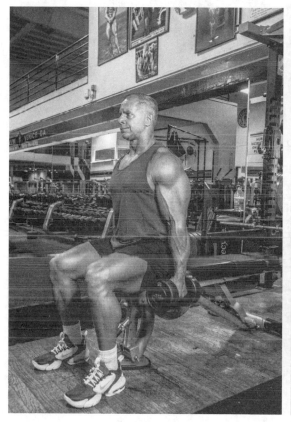 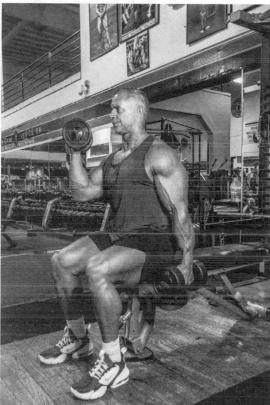

REVERSE GRIP BICEP CURL

With your palms facing down, grip an EZ curl bar and curl the weight up and then back down. Keep your elbows close to your torso.

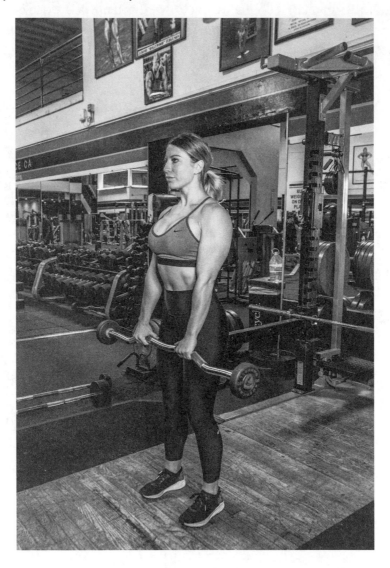

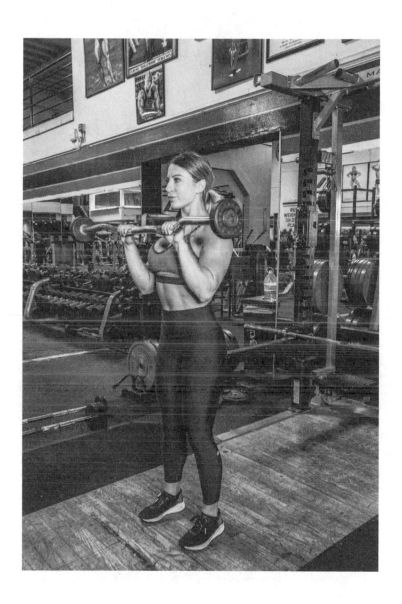

PULL-UP

Set your hands about shoulder width apart on a pull bar, using an overhand grip. Try to pull your chest to the bar or get your head above the bar.

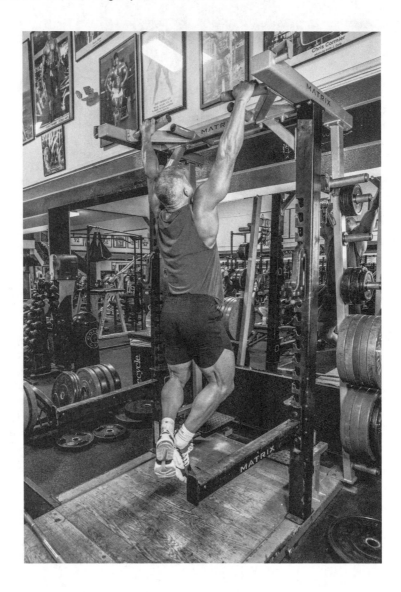

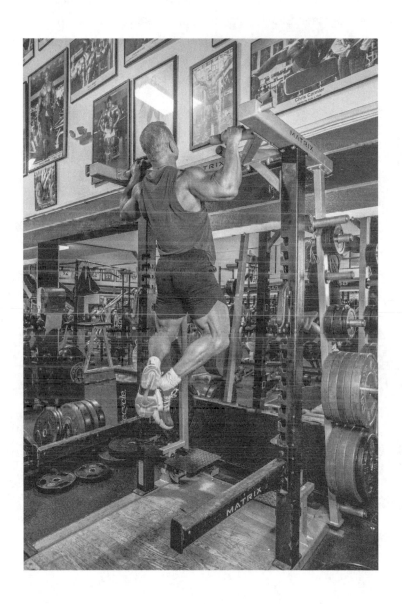

PULLDOWNS

Using a lat pulldown machine, grab the bar at the desired width, bring your torso back, and then pull the bar down until it touches your upper chest. Concentrate on squeezing your back muscles together. Slowly raise the bar back to the starting position. You can do this exercise with either an overhand grip or an underhand grip to work different muscles.

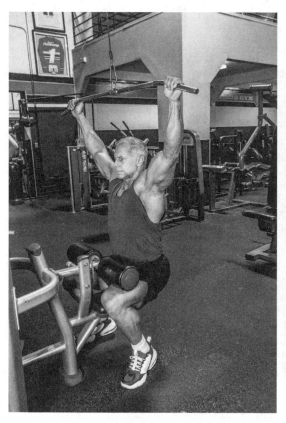 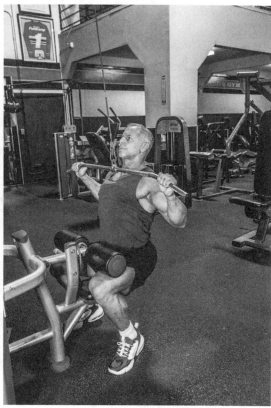

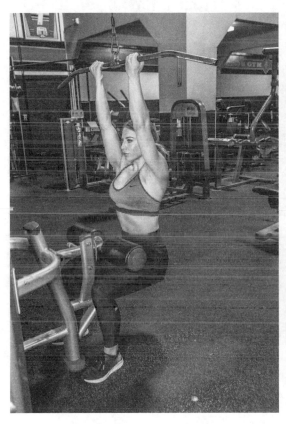 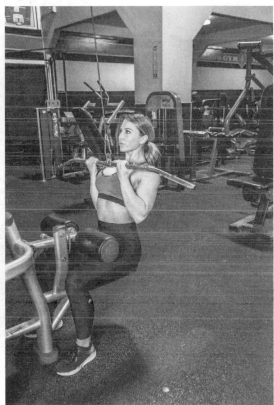

WRIST CURL

Holding dumbbells or a small barbell with palms facing up and forearms braced on a bench, curl the weight up and then down using your wrists.

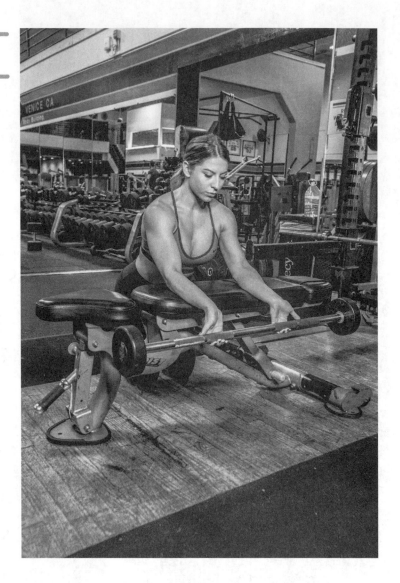

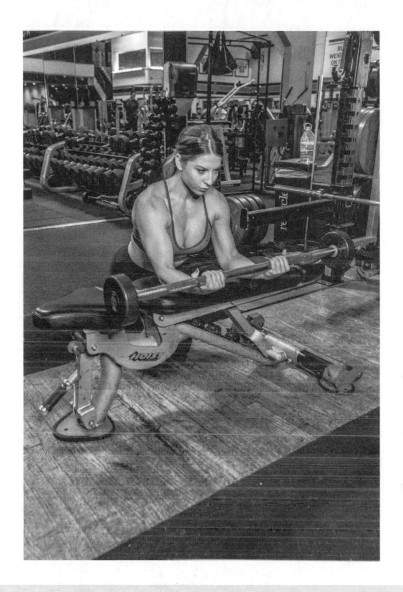

VARIATION (Not Pictured) HYPEREXTENSION

On a hyperextension bench, cross your arms in front of you or behind your head and bend forward at the waist as far as you can, keeping your back flat. Raise yourself back up and repeat. Use a weight plate for added difficulty.

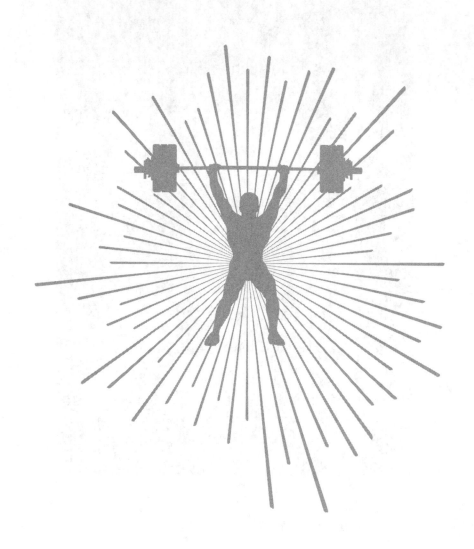

PLYOMETRICS

AIR SQUAT

This is very simple and is done without weights. With your hands in front of you, perform a squat, squatting to a point where your thighs are at least parallel to the floor.

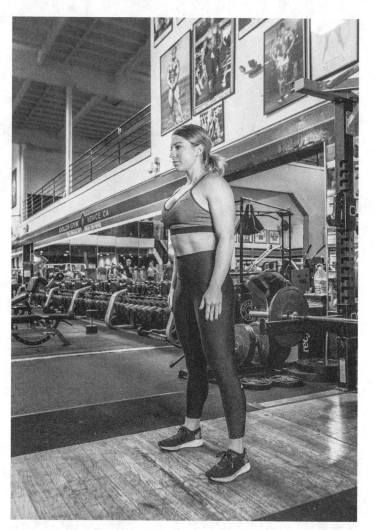

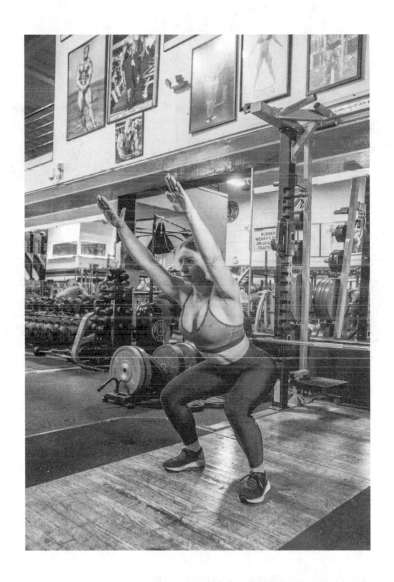

JUMP SQUAT

Perform the air squat but jump up out of the bottom position. Repeat as necessary.

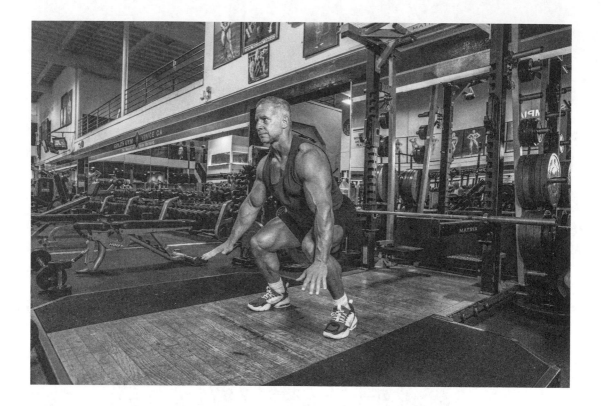

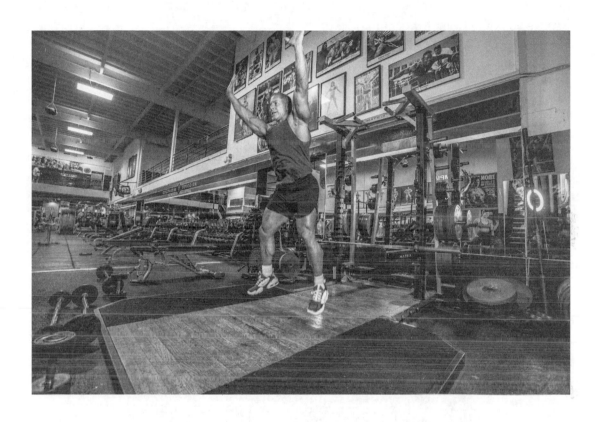

SINGLE-ARM DUMBBELL SNATCH

Holding a dumbbell in one hand between your legs, squat close to the floor. Use your hips to explode up to accelerate the weight up and get under it so that you can catch it above your head with a straight arm.

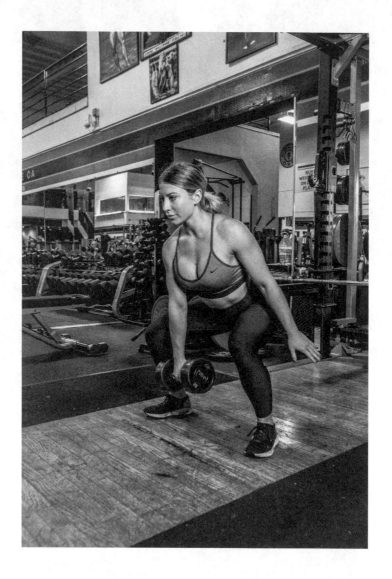

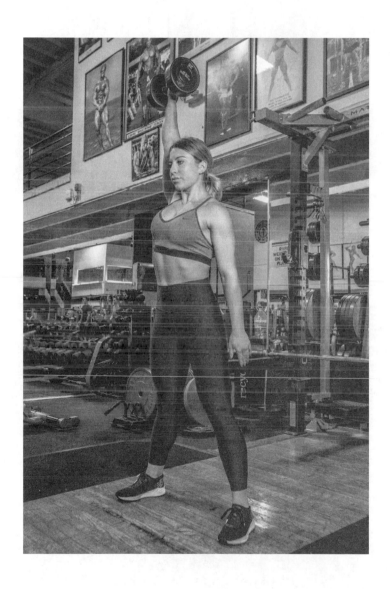

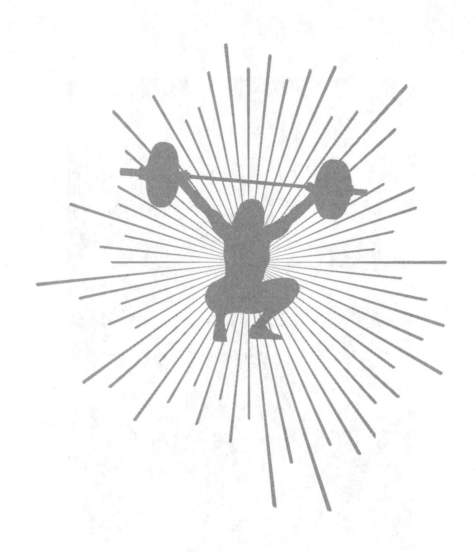

CARDIOVASCULAR EXERCISES

BURPEE

Stand with your feet shoulder width. Bend your knees and drop forward to place your hands on the floor. Kick your legs straight out behind you and immediately lower your entire body down to the ground, bending at the elbows. Then return to the squat position and explode up into the air. There are many variations on a burpee. Use one that works for you.

KETTLEBELL SWING

With your feet slightly wider than shoulder width, hold a kettlebell in front of your body. Brush your arms on your inner thighs extending your knees and hips while accelerating the kettlebell upward. Once the kettlebell is in the air, let it get to about shoulder height and then allow it to come back down before explosively driving it upward again.

MOUNTAIN CLIMBERS

Begin in a push-up position, with your weight supported by your hands and toes. Bring one leg up until it's under your hip and then move it back to the starting position. Do the same with the other leg. Explosively alternate bringing your legs up and back for the desired amount of time or reps.

ABS AND CORE

BUTTERFLY SIT-UP

Lying faceup on the ground with the soles of your feet pressed together, perform a sit-up and reach your hands toward your feet.

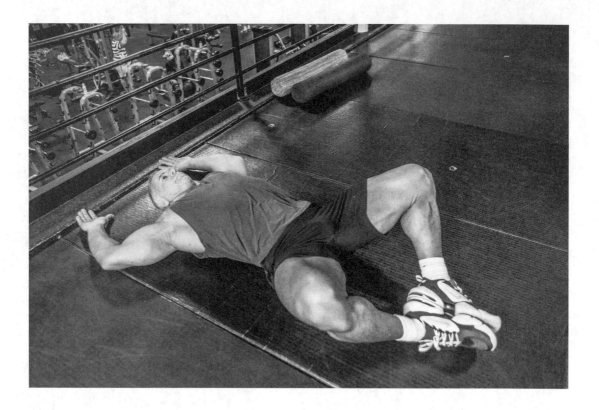

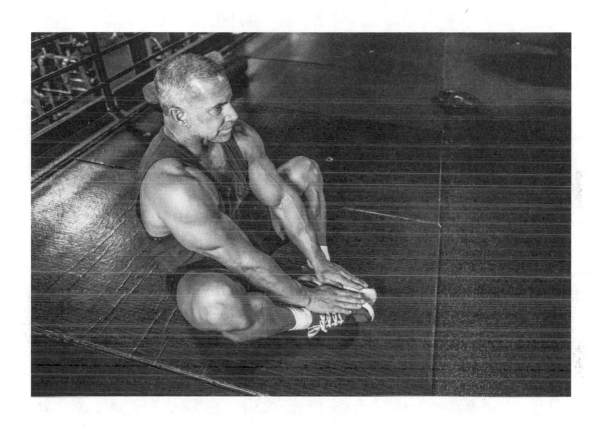

SIDE PLANK

Lie on one side, either on the floor or on a bench, with your legs on top of each other and fully extended. Using your lower elbow and forearm, press your body up, making sure to keep your abs tight. Your body should form a straight line from shoulders to ankles.

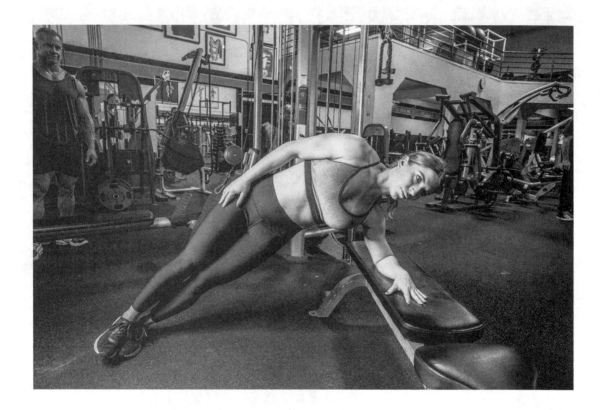

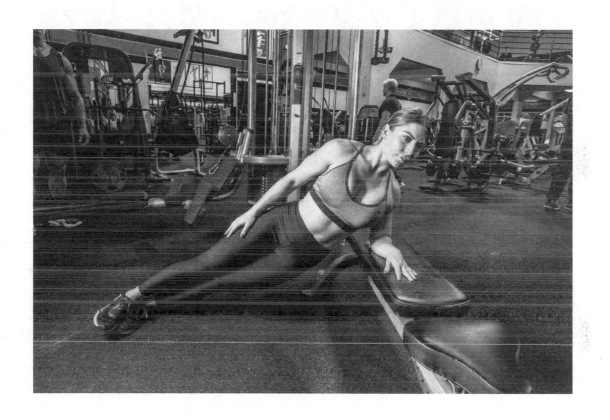

LEG LIFT

Sit on the floor with your legs straight and together. Lift your legs up and then lower them back down, making sure to keep your core tight. Keep lifting them up and down without touching the ground.

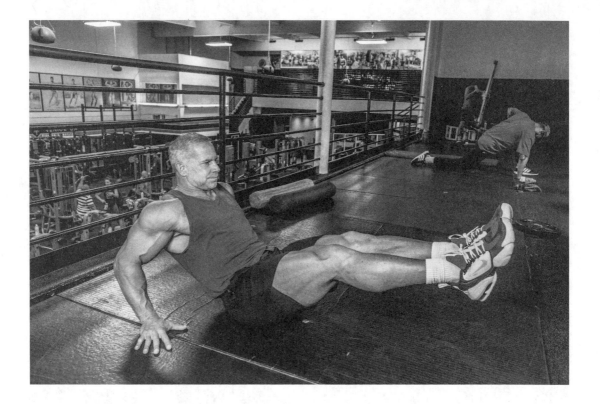

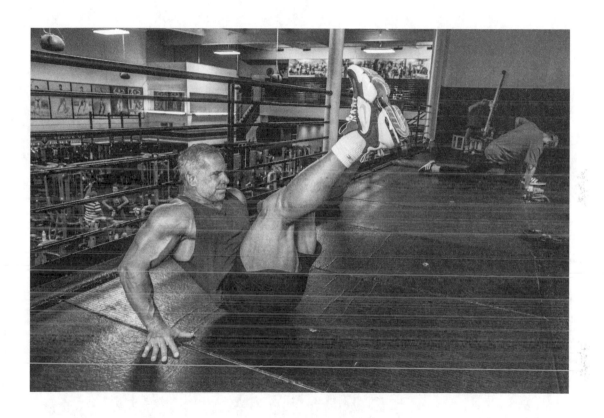

HEEL TOUCHES

Lie on the floor with knees bent and feet apart. Your arms should be extended by your side. Crunch up and forward over your torso about 3 to 4 inches to the right side, touching your right heel as you hold the contraction for a second. Then repeat to the left side.

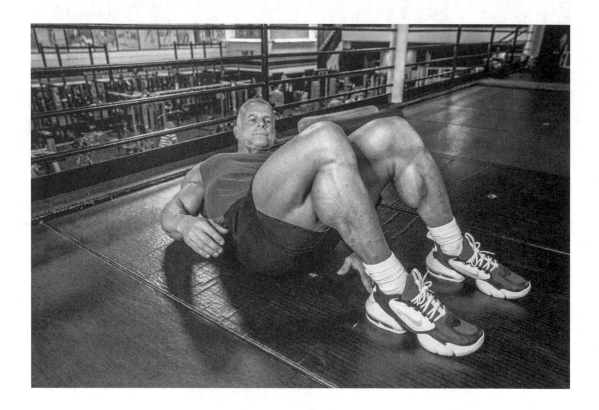

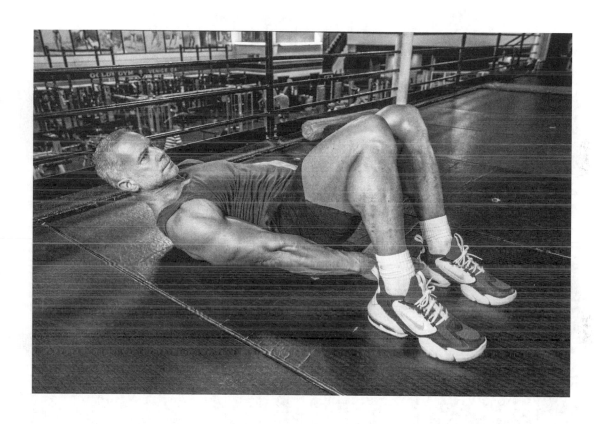

HANGING LEG RAISES

Hang from a chin-up bar with both arms extended. Exhaling, raise your legs until they are at a 90-degree angle to your torso. Hold the contraction for a second or so. If this version of the exercise is too hard, bend your knees and raise them until bent knees are at a 90-degree angle to your torso.

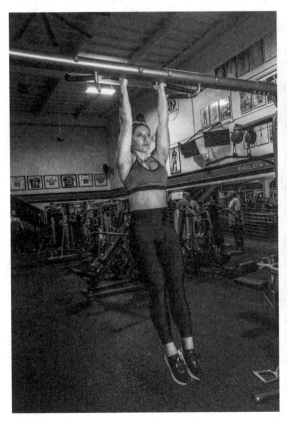
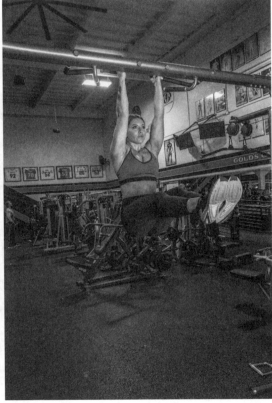

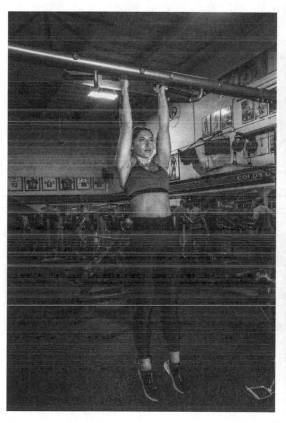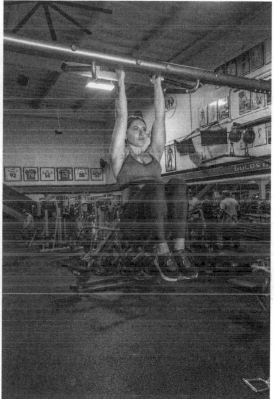

ATOMIC SIT-UP

Lie on your back with your hands outstretched behind you. Raise your feet 6 inches off the ground, keeping your legs slightly bent. Perform a sit-up, trying to reach your toes.

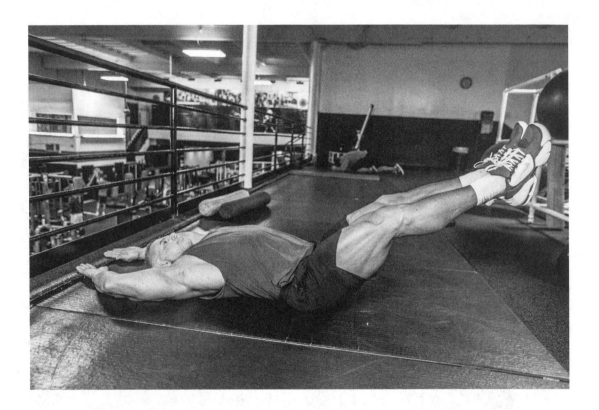

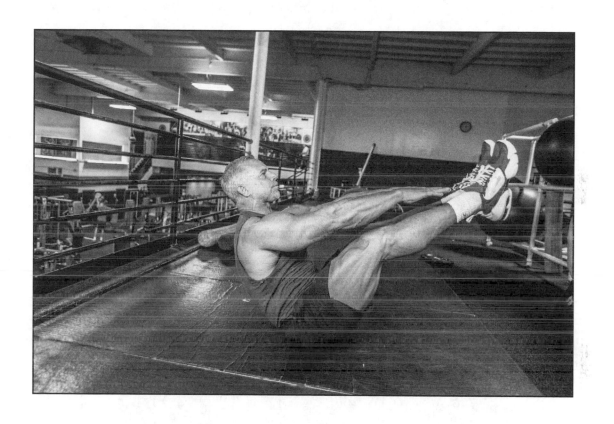

SEATED TWIST

Sitting on the floor with your knees bent and legs raised, lean back while keeping your core tight and your head and hips still. Holding your hands together, twist first to your left and then to your right, going as far as your range of motion allows. If you want more intensity, you can hold a medicine ball in your hands as you twist left and right.

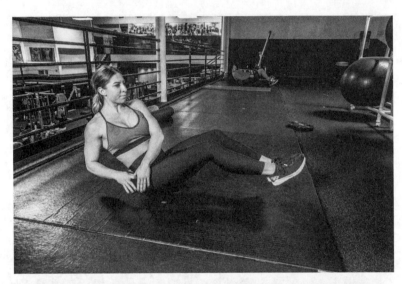

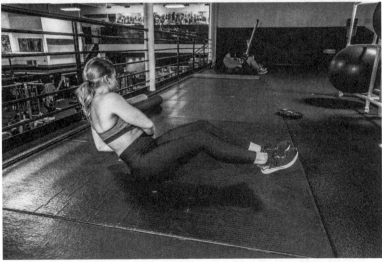

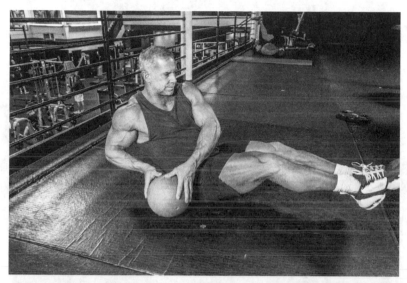

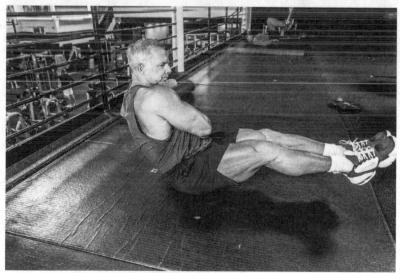

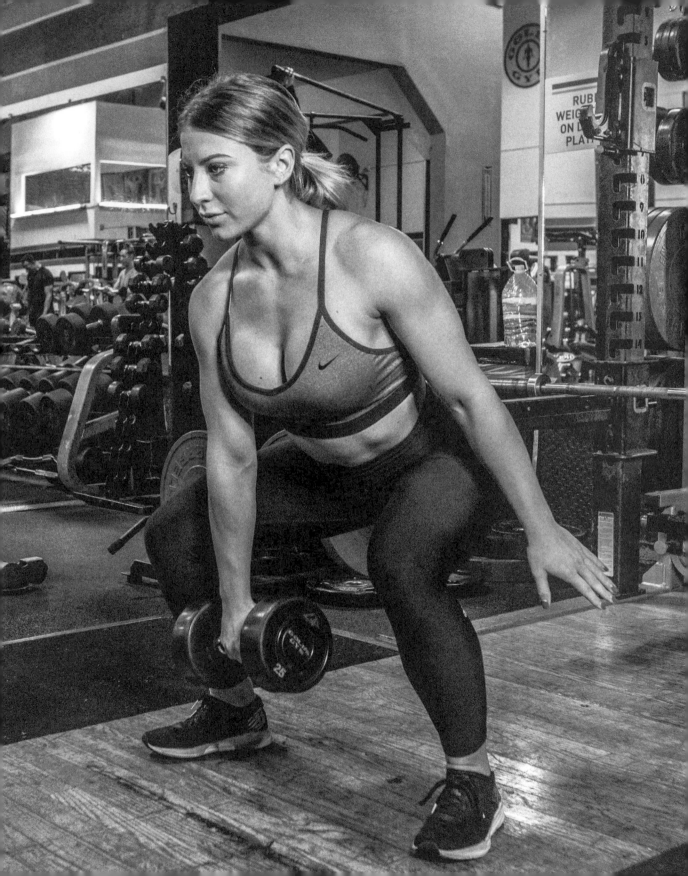

5

12 Weeks to Superhero Fit Workout

There's no secret formula. I lift heavy, work hard, and aim to be the best.
—Ronnie Coleman, eight-time Mr. Olympia

If you were ever to train with me, this is what we would do in actual week 1 so I can gauge where you are at. This is so you could measure for yourself and have a place to start from. It gives you a baseline you can come back to time and again to compare how much you accomplished and how much you improved from the first time you did it.

MONDAY, DAY 1

Welcome to it. You're about to jump into a workout that most of my clients have done. Do 1 pull-up, 2 dips, 3 push-ups, 4 sit-ups, and 5 squats, then 2 pull-ups, 4 dips, etc.... Work your way as far up and back down as you can. If you need to break some of the sets up (instead of 10 pull-ups you needed to break that set into 6, 3, 1 pull-ups) do so but when you find yourself needing to break up 2 or 3 of the exercises then start back down. In a perfect world you'll make it all the way to 10, 20, 30, 40, 50 and back down to 1, 2, 3, 4, 5.

Keep track of how far you made it and how long it took you.

Pull-ups × 1, 2, 3, 4, 5, 6, 7, 8, 9, 10, 9, 8, 7, 6, 5, 4, 3, 2, 1

Dips × 2, 4, 6, 8, 10, 12, 14, 16, 18, 20, 18, 16, 14, 12, 10, 8, 6, 4, 2

Push-ups × 3, 6, 9, 12, 15, 18, 21, 24, 27, 30, 27, 24, 21, 18, 15, 12, 9, 6, 3

Sit-ups × 4, 8, 12, 16, 20, 24, 28, 32, 36, 40, 36, 32, 28, 24, 20, 16, 12, 8, 4

Squats ×5, 10, 15, 20, 25, 30, 35, 40, 45, 50, 45, 40, 35, 30, 25, 20, 15, 10, 5

TUESDAY, DAY 2: CARDIO LSD (LONG SLOW DISTANCE)

Use the 180 BPM (beats per minute) HR (heart rate) minus your age as a ballpark number. So if you are a thirty-year-old: 180 − 30 = 150. So you LSD HR window would be 140–150 BPM

Go for a run, bike, swim, elliptical, etc. Take your pick. Get your HR into the 140–150 BPM and live there for a while: 20 minutes, 30 minutes, 40 minutes. What have you got? What kind of time are you willing to invest?

WEDNESDAY, DAY 3

Off

THURSDAY, DAY 4

10-minute easy run

How strong are you? What kind of weight can you push/pull for these reps?

Squats __ × 20, __ × 15, __ × 15, __ × 15, __ × 15

Bench press __ × 20, __ × 15, __ ×1 2, __ × 10, __ × 8

Barbell bent row __ ×15, __ × 12, __ × 12, __ × 12, __ × 10

Pulldowns (wide grip) __ × 15, __ × 12, (reverse narrow grip) __ × 12, __ × 12, __ × 12

Abs 100 reps of any combination you choose)

FRIDAY, DAY 5

Jump rope 3 minutes

Shoulder press __ × 15, __ × 12, __ × 10, __ × 8, __ × 8

Upright rows __ × 15, __ × 15, __ × 12, , __ × 12, , __ × 10

Side lateral raises __ × 15, __ × 15, __ × 15, __ × 15

Standing calf raises __ × 20, __ × 20, __ × 20, __ × 20

SATURDAY, DAY 6

400-meters easy run

1-mile "timed" run

400-meters easy cool down/walk

SUNDAY, DAY 7

Off

MONDAY, DAY 8: LEGS AND ABS

Warm-up: 10-minute easy run

Leg extensions (to pre-exhaust the quads) __ × 20, __ × 15, __ × 15, __ × 15

Squats __ × 20, __ × 15, __ × 12, __ × 10, __ × 8, __ × 6

Leg presses __ × 20, __ × 12, __ × 12, __ × 12

Leg curls __ × 15, __ × 12, __ × 12, __ × 12

Calf raises __ × 20, __ × 20, __ × 20, __ × 20

Abs 1 round = (sit-ups × 25; crunches × 25; leg lifts × 25; heel touches × 25)

TUESDAY, DAY 9: BACK AND BICEPS

Warm-up: 5 pull-ups / 10 push-ups / 15 squats × 2

Pulldowns (wide grip) __ × 20, __ × 15, __ × 12; (reverse narrow grip) __ × 10, __ × 8, __ × 6, __ × 1RM

Dumbbell rows __ × 15, __ × 12, __ × 12, __ × 12

Barbell curls __ × 15, __ × 12, __ × 12, __ × 12, __ × 12

WEDNESDAY, DAY 10: CHEST AND TRICEPS

Warm-up: 10-minute easy run

Bench presses __ × 20, __ × 15, __ × 12, __ × 10, __ × 8

Dumbbell flyes __ × 15, __ × 15, __ × 15, __ × 15

Lying triceps extensions __ × 20, __ × 20, __ × 15, __ × 15, __ × 15

Dumbbell kickbacks __ × 15, __ × 15, __ × 15, __ × 15

THURSDAY, DAY 11: SHOULDERS AND ABS

Warm-up: 15 jumping jacks / arm circles forward and
backward

Standing presses (bar) __ × 15, __ × 12, __ × 10, __ × 8, __ × 8

Upright rows (bar) __ × 15, __ × 15, __ × 15, __ × 15

Dumbbell side lateral raises __ × 12, __ × 12, __ × 12, __ × 12

Abs 1 round = (side plank raises × 15L/15R;
hanging leg raises × 15; atomic sit-ups × 15; seated twists × 15)

FRIDAY, DAY 12: AMRAP (AS MANY ROUNDS AS POSSIBLE) DAY

Warm-up: 10-minute easy run

Old favorite: CrossFit Cindy = 5 pull-ups, 10 push-ups, 15 squats
AMRAP in 20 minutes. If you can't; do 20 minutes, try 15, but
don't stop—no phone, no chitchat, just ready, set, go!

SATURDAY, DAY 13: LSD (LONG SLOW DISTANCE)

Go jog, swim, bike, or row, but go longer than your last LSD
day.

SUNDAY, DAY 14

Rest

WEEK 3

MONDAY, DAY 15: LEGS AND ABS

Warm-up: 10-minute easy run

Leg extensions (to pre-exhaust the quads) __ × 20, __ × 15, __ × 15, __ × 15

Squats __ × 20, __ × 20, __ × 20, __ × 20, __ × 20

Leg presses __ × 15, __ × 12, __ × 10, __ × 8

Leg curls __ × 10, __ × 8, __ × 8, __ × 8

Calf raises __ × 20, __ × 20, __ × 20, __ × 20

Abs 2 rounds = (sit-ups × 25; crunches × 25; leg lifts × 25; heel touches × 25). How many rounds can you do? More than last week, I hope!

TUESDAY, DAY 16: BACK AND BICEPS

Warm-up: 5 pull-ups / 10 push-ups / 15 squats × 2

Pulldowns (wide grip) __ × 20, __ × 15, __ × 15, __ × 15, __ × 12, __ × 10

Dumbbell rows __ × 15, __ × 12, __ × 10, __ × 8

Barbell curls __ × 15, __ × 12, __ × 10, __ × 8, __ × 6, __ × 15

WEDNESDAY, DAY 17: CHEST AND TRICEPS

Warm-up: 5 pull-ups / 10 push-ups / 15 squats × 2

Bench presses __ × 20, __ × 15, __ × 15, __ × 15, __ × 12

Dumbbell flyes __ × 15, __ × 12, __ × 10, __ × 10

Lying triceps extensions __ × 20, __ × 15, __ × 12, __ × 10, __ × 10

Dumbbell kickbacks __ × 15, __ × 15, __ × 15, __ × 15

THURSDAY, DAY 18: SHOULDERS AND ABS

Standing presses __ × 15, __ × 15, __ × 12, __ × 12, __ × 10

Upright rows __ × 15, __ × 12 __ × 10, __ × 10

Side lateral raises __ × 15, __ × 12, __ × 10, __ × 8

Abs 2 rounds = (side plank raises × 15L/15R; hanging leg raises × 15; atomic sit-ups × 15; seated twists × 15)

FRIDAY, DAY 19: LSD (LONG SLOW DISTANCE)

Go jog, swim, bike, row, or a combination of these. Go a bit longer than last week, but you'll want fairly fresh legs for tomorrow.

SATURDAY, DAY 20

400 meters easy

2-mile timed run

400 meters easy cooldown / walk

SUNDAY, DAY 21

Easy active recovery day. Whatever you didn't do yesterday—run, swim, bike—go do it and be easy about it. All you want is to break a light sweat and get the blood flowing through your muscles to aid in their recovery. Choose an activity you can drag the kids along for.

WEEK 4

Is exactly the same as Week 2, but I want MORE. More weight, an extra rep wherever you can get one or do the same of everything in less time.

MONDAY, DAY 22: LEGS AND ABS

Warm-up: 10-minute easy run

Leg extensions (to pre-exhaust the quads) __ × 20, __ × 15, __ × 15, __ × 15

Squats __ × 20, __ × 15, __ × 12, __ × 10, __ × 8, __ × 6

Leg presses __ × 20, __ × 12, __ × 12, __ × 12

Leg curls __ × 15, __ × 12, __ × 12, __ × 12

Calf raises __ × 20, __ × 20, __ × 20, __ × 20

Abs 2 rounds = (sit-ups × 25; crunches × 25; leg lifts × 25; heel touches × 25) How many rounds can you do?

TUESDAY, DAY 23: BACK AND BICEPS

Warm-up: 5 pull-ups / 10 push-ups / 15 squats × 2

Pulldowns (wide grip) __ × 20, __ × 15, __ × 12; (reverse narrow grip) __ × 10, __ × 8, __ × 6, __ × 1RM

Dumbbell rows __ × 15, __ × 12, __ × 12, __ × 12

Barbell curls __ × 15, __ × 12, __ × 12, __ × 12, __ × 12

WEDNESDAY, DAY 24: CHEST AND TRICEPS

Warm-up: 5 pull-ups / 10 push-ups / 15 squats × 2

Bench presses __ × 20, __ × 15, __ × 12, __ × 10, __ × 8

Dumbbell flyes __ × 15, __ × 15, __ × 15, __ × 15

Lying triceps extensions __ × 20, __ × 20, __ × 15, __ × 15, __ × 15

Dumbbell kickbacks __ × 15, __ × 15, __ × 15, __ × 15

THURSDAY, DAY 25: SHOULDERS AND ABS

Standing presses __ × 15, __ × 12, __ × 10, __ × 8, __ × 8

Upright rows __ × 15, __ × 15, __ × 15, __ × 15

Side lateral raises __ × 12, __ × 12, __ × 12, __ × 12

Abs 2 rounds = (side plank raises × 15L / 15R; hanging leg raises × 15; atomic sit-ups × 15; seated twist × 15)

FRIDAY, DAY 26: AMRAP (AS MANY ROUNDS AS POSSIBLE) DAY

Old favorite: CrossFit Cindy = 5 pull-ups, 10 push-ups, 15 squats AMRAP in 20 minutes. If you can't do 20 minutes, try 15, but don't stop—no phone, no chitchat.

SATURDAY, DAY 27: LSD (LONG SLOW DISTANCE)

Go jog, swim, bike, row, etc.

SUNDAY, DAY 28

Rest

Week 5 is exactly the same as Week 3, but I want MORE. More weight, an extra rep wherever you can get one or do the same of everything in less time.

MONDAY, DAY 29: LEGS AND ABS

Warm-up: 10-minute easy run

Leg extensions (to pre-exhaust the quads) __ × 20, __ × 15, __ × 15, __ × 15

Squats (The weight you choose here should be doable for the first set, difficult for the second set, and nearly unbearable by set 5.) __ × 20, __ × 20, __ × 20, __ × 20, __ × 20

Leg presses __ × 15, __ × 12, __ × 10, __ × 8

Leg curls __ × 10, __ × 8, __ × 8, __ × 8

Calf raises __ × 20, __ × 20, __ × 20, __ × 20, __ × 20

Abs 2 rounds = (sit-ups × 25; crunches × 25; leg lifts × 25; heel touches × 25)

TUESDAY, DAY 30: BACK AND BICEPS

Warm-up: 5 pull-ups / 10 push-ups / 15 squats × 2

Pulldowns (wide grip)__ × 20, __ × 15, __ × 15; (reverse narrow grip) __ × 15, __ × 12, __ × 10

Dumbbell rows (heavy)__ × 15, __ × 12, __ × 10, __ × 8

Barbell curls __ × 15, __ × 12, __ × 10, __ × 8, __ × 6, __ × 15

WEDNESDAY, DAY 31: LSD (LONG SLOW DISTANCE)

Swim, bike, run, or row. No running tomorrow, so go long!

THURSDAY, DAY 32: CHEST AND TRICEPS

Warm-up: 5 pull-ups / 10 push-ups / 15 squats x 2

Bench presses __ × 20, __ × 15, __ × 15, __ × 15, __ × 12

Dumbbell flyes __ × 15, __ × 12, __ × 10, __ × 10

Lying triceps extensions __ × 20, __ × 15, __ × 12, __ × 10, __ × 10

Dumbbell kickbacks __ × 15, __ × 15, __ × 15, __ × 15

FRIDAY, DAY 33: SHOULDERS AND ABS

Standing presses __ × 15, __ × 15, __ × 12, __ × 12, __ × 10

Upright rows __ × 15, __ × 12 __ × 10, __ × 10

Side lateral raises __ × 15, __ × 12, __ × 10, __ × 8

Abs 2 rounds = (side plank raises × 15L/15R; hanging leg raises × 15; atomic sit-ups × 15; seated twists × 15)

SATURDAY, DAY 34

Run 400 meters easy

2-mile timed run

400 meters easy cooldown / walk

SUNDAY, DAY 35: EASY ACTIVE RECOVERY DAY

Whatever you didn't do yesterday—run, swim, bike—go do it and be easy about it. All you want is to break a light sweat and get the blood flowing through your muscles to aid in their recovery.

WEEK 6

MONDAY, DAY 36

Welcome back. Let's see if you've improved. Do 1 pull-up, 2 dips, 3 push-ups, 4 sit-ups, and 5 squats, then 2 pull-ups, 4 dips, and so forth. Work your way as far up and down as you can. If you need to break up some of the sets (instead of doing 10 pull-ups, you needed to break that set into 6, 3, 1 pull-ups), do so, but when you find yourself needing to break up two or three of the exercises, then start back down. In a perfect world you'll make it all the way to 10, 20, 30, 40, 50 and back down to 1, 2, 3, 4, 5. Keep track of how far you made it and how long it took you. I hope you get further into it or complete it faster.

Pull-ups × 1, 2, 3, 4, 5, 6, 7, 8, 9, 10, 9, 8, 7, 6, 5, 4, 3, 2, 1

Dips × 2, 4, 6, 8, 10, 12, 14, 16, 18, 20, 18, 16, 14, 12, 10, 8, 6, 4, 2

Push-ups × 3, 6, 9, 12, 15, 18, 21, 24, 27, 30, 27, 24, 21, 18, 15, 12, 9, 6, 3

Sit-ups × 4, 8, 12, 16, 20, 24, 28, 32, 36, 40, 36, 32, 28, 24, 20, 16, 12, 8, 4

Squats × 5, 10, 15, 20, 25, 30, 35, 40, 45, 50, 45, 40, 35, 30, 25, 20, 15, 10, 5

TUESDAY, DAY 37: CARDIO LSD (LONG SLOW DISTANCE)

Use that 180 BPM (beats per minute) heart rate minus your age as a ballpark number. Thus if you are a thirty-year-old: 180 − 30 = 150. So your LSD heart rate window would be 140–150 BPM. Go for a run, bike, swim, use the elliptical, etc. Or choose a combination of two or more. Take your pick. Get your HR (heart rate) into the 140–150 BPM and live there for a while: 20 minutes, 30 minutes, 40 minutes. What have you got? What kind of time are you willing to invest?

WEDNESDAY, DAY 38

6 rounds of

Run 400 meters

Pull-ups 10

Push-ups 15

Squats 20

Sit-ups 20

Dips 12

Dumbbell curls __ × 12

Row 400 meters

Keep track of your times!

THURSDAY, DAY 39

How strong are you? What kind of weight can you push/pull for these reps? You did more work this week than you did in Week 1, but you can still manage more weight or more reps. You are capable of this. Look at Week 1's numbers; then beat them!

Squats __ × 20, __ × 15, __ × 15, __ × 15, __ × 15

Bench presses __ × 20, __ × 15, __ × 12, __ × 10, __ × 8

Barbell bent rows __ × 15, __ × 12, __ × 12, __ × 12, __ × 10

Pulldowns __ × 15, __ × 12, __ × 12, __ × 12, __ × 12

Abs 200 reps of any combination you choose

FRIDAY, DAY 40

Same as yesterday. You're looking to beat your Week 1 numbers. More weight or more reps or less time.

Jump rope 3 minutes

Shoulder presses __ × 15, __ × 12, __ × 10, __ × 8, __ × 8

Upright rows __ × 15, __ × 15, __ × 12, __ × 12, __ × 10

Side lateral raises __ × 15, __ × 15, __ × 15, __ × 15

Calf raises __ × 20, ___ × 20, ___ × 20, __ × 20

SATURDAY, DAY 41: FARTLEK RUN

Think of this as an LSD run with speed intervals spread intermittently throughout. Go on a LSD run, and after you're in your groove, race half a block to a lamppost or object. Once you get there, resume your LSD pace until you've pretty much gotten your breath back. Then pick out another marker up the road and sprint to it. Repeat this process for half of your normal LSD distance.

SUNDAY, DAY 42

Take a well-deserved day off.

WEEK 7

MONDAY, DAY 43: LEGS AND ABS

Your weights should be going up!

Warm up: 10-minute run

Leg extensions (to pre-exhaust the quads) __ × 20, __ × 15, __ × 15, __ × 15

Squats __ × 20, __ × 15, __ × 12, __ × 12, __ × 12

Leg presses (heavy) __ × 15, __ × 8, __ × 8, __ × 8__ × 8

Leg curls __ × 10, __ × 8, __ × 8, __ × 8, __ × 8, __ × 15 (After your last set of 8, pick a lighter weight and knock out another 15 reps.)

Walking lunges __ × 15, __ × 15, __ × 12, __ × 10 (steps each leg)

Abs 3 rounds = (sit-ups × 25, crunches × 25, leg lifts × 25, heel touches × 25). How many rounds can you do? More than last week, I hope!

TUESDAY, DAY 44: BACK AND SHOULDERS

Warm-up: 5 pull-ups / 10 push-ups / 15 squats × 2

Superset

Pulldowns (wide grip)__ × 20, __ × 15, __ × 15; (reverse narrow grip) __ × 12, __ × 10, __ × 8

Shoulder presses __ × 15, __ × 12, __ × 10, __ × 8, __ × 6, __ × 4

Dumbbell rows __ × 12, __ × 12, __ × 12, __ × 12

Side lateral raises ___ × 15, ___ × 12, ___ × 12, ___ × 10

Calf raises ___ × 20, ___ × 20, ___ × 20, ___ × 20, ___ × 20

WEDNESDAY, DAY 45: CHEST, BICEPS, AND TRICEPS

Warm-up (5 pull-ups / 10 push-ups / 15 squats) × 2

Superset

Bench presses ___ × 20, ___ × 20, ___ × 15, ___ × 15, ___ × 12

Alternating seated dumbbell curls ___ × 15, ___ × 15, ___ × 15, ___ × 12, ___ × 10

Superset

Standing triceps extension ___ × 20, ___ × 15, ___ × 12, ___ × 10, ___ × 8

Barbell curls ___ × 15, ___ × 15, ___ × 15, ___ × 12, ___ × 10

Abs (sit-ups × 25; crunches × 25; leg lifts × 25; heel touches × 25) How many rounds can you do? Three, four? More?

THURSDAY, DAY 46: CARDIO LSD (LONG SLOW DISTANCE)

Use that 180 BPM (beats per minute) heart rate (HR) minus your age as a ballpark number. Thus if you are a thirty-year-old: 180 − 30 = 150. So your LSD heart rate window would be 140–150 BPM. Go for a run, bike, swim, use the elliptical, etc. Or choose a combination of two or more. Take your pick. Get your HR into the 140–150 BPM and live there for a while: 20 minutes, 30 minutes, 40 minutes. You're coming up on Week 8 of a 12-week program. Before you know it, this 12 weeks is going to be over and you're going to look back and think *I could have done more*, so just go ahead and do more right now.

FRIDAY, DAY 47

It's on now!

Warm-up: 10-minute easy run and 5 pull-ups / 10 push-ups / 15 squats × 2. Oh, shit!

5 rounds of

30 sit-ups

10 dumbbell power snatches (in some circles men use a 50-pound dumbbell and women use a 35-pound dumbbell). For time, keep track of how long it takes you to pull this off.

SATURDAY, DAY 48: TIMED RUN

400 meters easy

3-mile timed run

400 meters easy cooldown / walk

SUNDAY, DAY 49

Day off

WEEK 8

MONDAY, DAY 50

Warm-up: 5 pull-ups / 10 push-ups / 15 squats × 3

Superset

Pulldowns __ × 20, __ × 15, __ × 15, __ × 12, __ × 10, __ × 8

Shoulder presses __ × 15, __ × 12, __ × 10, __ × 8, __ × 6, __ × 4

Dumbbell rows __ × 12, __ × 12, __ × 12, __ × 12

Side lateral raises __ × 15, __ × 12, __ × 12, __ × 10

Calf raises __ × 20, __ × 20, __ × 20, __ × 20, __ × 20

Abs 3 rounds = (sit-ups × 25; crunches × 25; leg lifts × 25; heel touches × 25)

TUESDAY, DAY 51

Warm-up: 5 pull-ups / 10 push-ups / 15 squats × 3

Superset

Bench presses __ × 20, __ × 20, __ × 15, __ × 15, __ × 12

Alternating seated dumbbell curls __ × 15, __ × 15, __ × 15, __ × 12, __ × 10

Superset

Standing triceps extensions __ × 20, __ × 15, __ × 12, __ × 10,
__ × 8

Barbell curls __ × 15, __ × 15, __ × 15, __ × 12, __ × 10

WEDNESDAY, DAY 52

400-meter run

50 burpees

400-meter run

30 burpees

400-meter run

20 burpees

400-meter run

All done for time

THURSDAY, DAY 53

Shoulder complex = 15 side lateral raises, 15 alternate front
lateral raises, 15 bent-over rear lateral raises, 15 overhead
presses, 15 upright rows. Do not put the weights down
until you've finished all five exercises. You can rest, but rest
with those dumbbells in your hands. Now pick up a slightly
heavier weight and do it again for sets of 12, then slightly
more weight for a set of 10, 8, 6.

Calf raises __ × 20, __ × 20, __ × 20, __ × 20, __ × 20

Abs 3 rounds = (sit-ups × 25; crunches × 25; leg lifts × 25;
heel touches × 25)

FRIDAY, DAY 54

400 meters easy

3-mile timed run

400 meters easy cooldown / walk

SATURDAY, DAY 55: LSD (LONG SLOW DISTANCE)

Run, swim, bike, row, or a combination of all. Tomorrow is a day
off, so put on some headphones and go big. Not fast. Go long.

SUNDAY, DAY 56

Day off

WEEK 9

MONDAY, DAY 57

Warm-up: 5 pull-ups / 10 push-ups / 15 squats × 3

Superset

Pulldowns __ × 20, __ × 15, __ × 12, __ × 10, __ × 8, __ × 6

Shoulder presses __ × 15, __ × 15, __ × 12, __ × 12, __ × 12

Dumbbell rows __ × 12, __ × 10, __ × 8, __ × 8, __ × 8

Side lateral raises __ × 15, __ × 12, __ × 12, __ × 10

Calf raises __ × 20, __ × 20, __ × 20, __ × 20, __ × 20

Abs 3 rounds = (sit-ups × 25; crunches × 25; leg lifts × 25;
heel touches × 25)

TUESDAY, DAY 58

1-mile easy run

Warm-up: 5 pull-ups / 10 push-ups / 15 squats × 3

Superset

Bench presses __ × 15, __ × 12, __ × 10, __ × 8, __ × 6, __ × 4

Alternating seated dumbbell curls __ × 15, __ × 15, __ × 15, __ × 12, __ × 10, __ × 8

Superset

Standing triceps extensions __ × 20, __ × 15, __ × 15, __ × 15, __ × 15

Alternating seated dumbbell curls __ × 15, __ × 15, __ × 15, __ × 12, __ × 10

WEDNESDAY, DAY 59

Run 800-meter easy warm-up, 1 mile quick pace

Sprint 2 × 800 meters / 2 × 400 meters / 4 ×100 meters

800-meter cooldown

THURSDAY, DAY 60

Day off

FRIDAY, DAY 61: AMRAP

She's back!

Warm-up: 10-minute easy run

CrossFit Cindy = 5 pull-ups, 10 push-ups, 15 squats AMRAP in 20 minutes

SATURDAY, DAY 62: LSD (LONG SLOW DISTANCE)

Go jog, swim, bike, or row, but you should be crushing your
Weeks 1 and 2 distances or times.

SUNDAY, DAY 63

Wrist curls __ × 20, __ × 15, __ × 15, __ × 12

Calf raises __ × 20, __ × 20, __ × 20, __ × 20

Abs 4 rounds = (sit-ups × 25; crunches × 25; leg lifts × 25;
heel touches × 25)

Easy day

WEEK 10

MONDAY, DAY 64: LSD (LONG SLOW DISTANCE)

Go jog, swim, bike, or row, but don't kill yourself.

TUESDAY, DAY 65

CrossFit Murph* (You had to know this was coming at some
point.)

1-mile run

100 pull-ups / 200 push-ups / 300 squats (in any order
you'd like)

1-mile run

For time!

---

* Murph is a classic CrossFit workout known as a Hero WOD (workout of the day), made to
honor the men and women who have fallen in the line of duty. It was named after Navy lieutenant
Michael Murphy, who was killed in Afghanistan on June 28, 2005.

WEDNESDAY, DAY 66

Day off

THURSDAY, DAY 67

6 rounds of

Run 400 meters

Pull-ups 10

Push-ups 15

Squats 20

Sit-ups 20

Dips 12

Dumbbell curls __ × 12

Row 400 meters

You better beat your Week 6 numbers.

FRIDAY, DAY 68

Wrist curls __ × 20, __ × 15, __ × 15, __ × 12

Calf raises __ × 20, __ × 20, __ × 20, __ × 20

Abs 4 rounds = (sit-ups × 25; crunches × 25; leg lifts × 25; heel touches × 25)

Easy day

SATURDAY, DAY 69

400 meters easy

4-mile timed run

400 meters easy cooldown / walk

SUNDAY, DAY 70

Day off

WEEK 11

MONDAY, DAY 71

1-mile easy run

Warm-up: 5 pull-ups / 10 push-ups / 15 squats × 4

Superset (8 set × 8 reps)

Dumbbell rows __ × 8, __ × 8, __ × 8, __ × 8, __ × 8, __ × 8, __ × 8, __ × 8

Dumbbell bench presses __ × 8, __ × 8, __ × 8, __ × 8, __ × 8, __ × 8, __ × 8, __ × 8

Abs 3 rounds = (sit-ups × 25; crunches × 25; leg lifts × 25; heel touches × 25)

TUESDAY, DAY 72

1-mile easy run

Warm-up: 5 pull-ups / 10 push-ups / 15 squats × 4

Shoulder complex = 15 side lateral raises, 15 alternate front lateral raises, 15 bent-over rear lateral raises, 15 overhead presses, 15 upright rows. Do not put the weights down until you've finished all five exercises. You can rest, but rest with those dumbbells in your hands. Then pick up a slightly heavier weight and do it again for sets of 12, then slightly more weight for a set of 10, 8, 6.

Calf raises __ × 20, __ × 20, __ × 20, __ × 20, __ × 20

WEDNESDAY, DAY 73: BICEPS AND TRICEPS

Warm-up: 20 jumping jacks / arm circles forward and backward

Superset

Lying triceps extensions __ × 20, __ × 15, __ × 12, __ × 12, __ × 12

Standing alternating dumbbell curls __ × 20, __ × 15, __ × 12, __ × 10, __ × 10

Dumbbell kickbacks __ × 20, __ × 15, __ × 12, __ × 12, __ × 12

Reverse EZ bar curls __ × 15, __ × 15, __ × 15, __ × 15, __ × 15

Abs 4 rounds = (sit-ups × 25; crunches × 25; leg lifts × 25; heel touches × 25)

THURSDAY, DAY 74

Warm-up: 10-minute easy run and 5 pull-ups / 10 push-ups / 15 squats × 4. What? YES!

5 rounds of

30 sit-ups

10 dumbbell power snatches (in some circles, men use a 50-pound dumbbell and women use a 35-pound dumbbell)

For time, keep track of how long it takes you to pull this off.

FRIDAY, DAY 75

Warm-up: 1800-meter easy run, 1 mile quick pace

Sprint 2 × 800 meters / 2 × 400 meters / 4 × 100 meters

800-meter cooldown

SATURDAY, DAY 76: LSD (LONG SLOW DISTANCE)

Go jog, swim, bike, or row, but you should be crushing your Weeks 1 and 2 distances or times.

SUNDAY, DAY 77

Day off

WEEK 12

MONDAY, DAY 78

Welcome to it. So here we are back at the beginning. You know the drill. Let's see what you've got. All the way through it, bottom to top and back down as fast as you can pull it off. Keep track of how far you made it and how long it took you.

Pull-ups × 1, 2, 3, 4, 5, 6, 7, 8, 9, 10, 9, 8, 7, 6, 5, 4, 3, 2, 1

Dips × 2, 4, 6, 8, 10, 12, 14, 16, 18, 20, 18, 16, 14, 12, 10, 8, 6, 4, 2

Push-ups × 3, 6, 9, 12, 15, 18, 21, 24, 27, 30, 27, 24, 21, 18, 15, 12, 9, 6, 3

Sit-ups × 4, 8, 12, 16, 20, 24, 28, 32, 36, 40, 36, 32, 28, 24, 20, 16, 12, 8, 4

Squats × 5, 10, 15, 20, 25, 30, 35, 40, 45, 50, 45, 40, 35, 30, 25, 20, 15, 10, 5

TUESDAY, DAY 79: FARTLEK RUN 2

Think of it as an LSD run with speed intervals spread intermittently throughout. Go on an LSD run, and after you're in your grove, race half a block to a lamppost or object. Once you get there, resume your LSD pace until you've pretty much gotten your breath back. Then pick out another marker up the road and sprint to it. Repeat this process for half of your normal LSD distance.

WEDNESDAY, DAY 80

Warm up: 10-minute easy run

This is Week 1's workout, so I'll ask you again: What kind of weight can you push/pull for these reps?

Squats __ × 20, __ × 15, __ × 15, __ × 15, __ × 15

Bench presses __ × 20, __ × 15, __ × 12, __ × 10, __ × 8

Barbell bent rows __ × 15, __ × 12, __ × 12, __ × 12, __ × 10

Pulldowns (wide grip) __ × 15, __ × 12; (reverse narrow grip) __ × 12, __ × 12, __ × 12

Abs 3 rounds = (sit-ups × 25; crunches × 25; leg lifts × 25; heel touches × 25)

THURSDAY, DAY 81

Warm up: 800-meter run, 1 mile quick pace

Sprint 2 × 800 meters / 2 × 400 meters / 4 × 100 meters

800-meter cooldown

FRIDAY, DAY 82

Jump rope 5 minutes

Shoulder presses __ × 15, __ × 12, __ × 10, __ × 8, __ × 8

Upright rows __ × 15, __ × 15, __ × 12, __ × 12, __ × 10

Side lateral raises __ × 15, __ × 15, __ × 15, __ × 15

Standing calf raises __ × 20, __ × 20, __ × 20, __ × 20

SATURDAY, DAY 83

400 meters easy

1 mile timed run (at this point you should be hauling ass for a
1-mile run)

400 meters easy cooldown / walk

SUNDAY, DAY 84

Day off for the last time

Well done.

Whatever you did I hope you gave it your absolute best effort. That's
what my clients give. They give their all. They invest what they can, and
then they go on camera and it's captured for the world to see.

EXPERT TIPS

- Practice good form on every rep.
- Remember to approach each and every rep using the
  concentric and then eccentric portion on your lifts—hugely
  important so that you get the most out of every rep!
- Focus on what you are doing on every rep.
- If it's too intense, dial it down.
- Listen to yourself; if something doesn't feel right, stop.
- Remember to breathe.

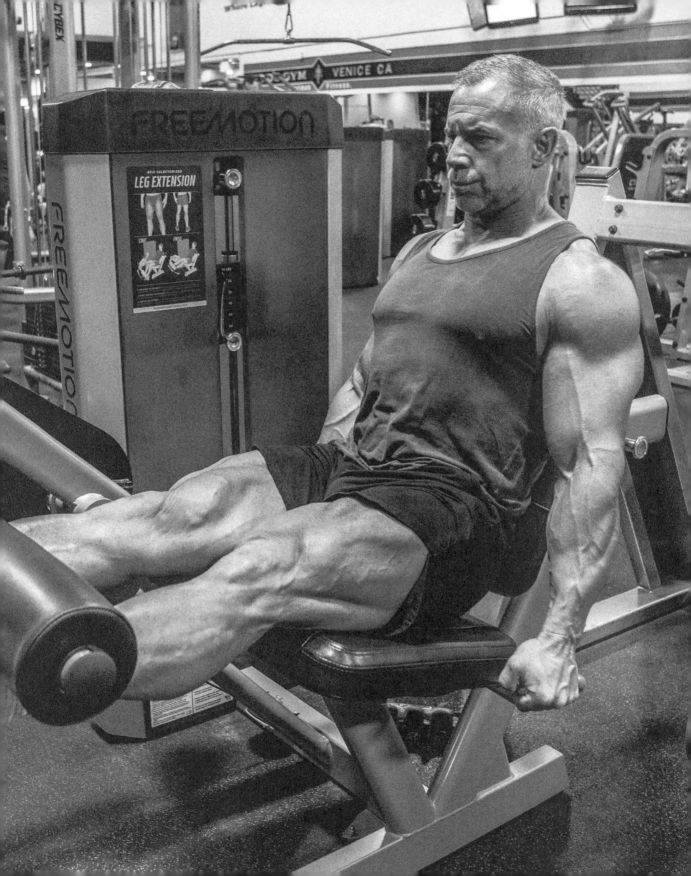

More Hero Workouts

I'm gonna do today what other people aren't willing to.
So I can do tomorrow what other people can't.

—Mat Fraser, four-time Fittest Man on Earth

T he main thing I want people to see from these workouts is that there is no secret. My clients do the same kind of things you would at the gym, but they do it with great effort and intensity.

I'll say this again because it bears repeating, I take pride in the fact that when I go to gyms with clients that after they've been working out a while, people start to watch. They do this not because it's this or that well-known person, but because they can't believe my clients are working as hard as they're working. That they're dripping sweat, out of breath, not talking, and they haven't stopped since we started.

BRAD PITT—JUNE 17, 2003

Leg day: Superset

Leg extensions 90 lb × 15, 15, 15, 15

Push-ups × 15, 12, 12, 12

Sit-ups × 15, 15, 15, 15

Squats 50 lb × 20, 135 lb × 15, 165 lb × 15, 185 lb × 15, 205 lb × 12, 225 lb × 10, 245 lb × 8

Leg presses 90 lb × 20, 140 lb × 20, 180 lb × 20, 180 lb × 20

Leg curls 60 lb × 15, 70 lb × 12, 70 lb × 12, 70 lb × 10, 70 lb × 10

Standing calf raises 100 lb × 20, 110 lb × 20, 120 lb × 18, 130 lb × 17

BRAD PITT—JUNE 23, 2006

Arms

Elliptical 10 minutes / level 8

Superset

Lying triceps extensions 35 lb × 15, 40 lb × 15, 45 lb × 12, 50 lb × 12, 55 lb × 10

Barbell curls 45 lb × 15, 50 lb × 12, 55 lb × 12, 55 lb × 12, 55 lb × 12

Hanging knee raises × 20, × 15, × 15, × 12, × 12

Superset

Standing triceps extensions 50 lb × 12, 55 lb × 12, 60 lb × 10, 60 lb × 10, 60 lb × 9

Seated dumbbell curls 20 lb × 15, 25 lb × 12, 30 lb × 10, 30 lb × 10, 30 lb × 10

ROW 1,500 meters 6:26

CHANNING TATUM/MARLON WAYANS—FEBRUARY 7, 2008

For time: pull-ups, dips, push-ups, sit-ups, squats ladder up and down

Pull-ups 1, 2, 3, 4, 5, 6, 7, 8, 9, 10, 9, 8, 7, / 6, 5, 4, 3, 2, 1

Dips 2, 4, 6, 8, 10, 12, 14, 16, 18, 20, 18, 16, 14, / 12, 10, 8, 6, 4, 2

Push-ups 3, 6, 9, 12, 15, 18, 21, 24, 27, 30, 27, 24, 21, / 18, 15, 12, 9, 6, 3

Sit-ups 4, 8, 12, 16, 20, 24, 28, 32, 36, 40, 36, 32, 28, / 24, 20, 16, 12, 8, 4

Squats 5, 10, 15, 20, 25, 30, 35, 40, 45, 50, 45, 40, 35, / 30, 25, 20, 15, 10, 5

Chan and Marlon's first time at this workout. They both made it to the round of 7s and back down. Marlon 39:25.81 / Channing 35:02.02.

CHANNING TATUM—AUGUST 6, 2010

For time:

Pull-ups × 100

Push-ups × 100

Sit-ups × 100

Squats × 100

Total time 23:38.05

CHANNING TATUM—AUGUST 18, 2010

6 rounds. Each round consists of:

Run 400 meters

Pull-ups × 12

Push-ups × 20

Squats × 25

Dips × 15

Curls 30 lb dumbbell × 12

Kettlebell swings 44 kg × 12

Sit-ups × 25

Times: Rd 1, 6:28; Rd 2, 7:21; Rd 3, 7:49; Rd 4, 7:49; Rd 5, 7:18; Rd 6, 7:05.

Total time 43:51.48

CHRIS HEMSWORTH—MARCH 14, 2011

Back and Biceps

Pulldowns Hammer Strength 90 lb × 20, 140 lb × 15, 180 lb × 15, 230 lb × 12, 270 lb × 10, 300 lb × 8

Dumbbell rows: 65 lb × 15, 70 lb × 15, 75 lb × 12, 80 lb × 10, 85 lb × 10, 90 lb × 10

Dumbbell curls: 30 lb × 15, 35 lb × 15, 40 lb × 15, 45 lb × 12, 50 lb × 10, 45 lb × 6, 40 lb × 6, 35 lb × 11, 30 lb × 15

Hyperextensions: × 15, 15, 15

Abs (sit-ups × 25; crunches × 25; seated twists with 10 lb ball × 25) × 4 rounds

ALICE EVE—DECEMBER 21, 2017

4 rounds for time

Run 800 meters, 600 meters, 400 meters, 200 meters

Assisted pull-ups 50 lb × 15, 12, 10, 8

Push-ups × 25, 20, 15, 10

Sit-ups × 25, 20, 15, 12

Crunches × 25, 25, 25, 25

Squats × 25, 25, 25, 25

Dumbbell curls 12 lb × 15, 12, 10, 8

Dumbbell kickbacks 12 lb × 15, 12, 10, 8

Mountain climbers × 12, 10, 8, 6

ROW × 500 meters, 400 meters, 300 meters, 200 meters

Total time 43:38.38

EMORY COHEN—JANUARY 18, 2018

Row 1,400 meters = 6:00

8 rounds of

Pull-ups × 3

Push-ups × 8

Sit-ups × 12

Squats × 12

Total time 9:55.70

Superset 10 sets for 10 reps

Dumbbell rows 40 lb × 10, 10, 10, 10, 10, 10, 10, 10, 10, 10

Dumbbell bench presses 40 lb × 10, 10, 10, 10, 10, 10, 10, 10, 10, 10

Pulldowns 125 lb × 12, 12, 12, 12, 12

AUGUSTO AGUILERA—JANUARY 26, 2018

Murph:

1-mile run 7:14.28

100 pull-ups

200 push-ups

300 squats

26:54.38

1-mile run 11:52.22

Total time 46:00.89

COREY HAWKINS—AUGUST 30, 2018

Row 1,100 meters: 4:29.0

Pull-ups × 13, 10, 8, 8

Push-ups × 15, 12, 10, 10

Squats × 15, 12, 10, 10

Pulldowns (wide grip) 95 lb × 15, 110 lb × 12; (medium width) 125 lb × 10, 125 lb × 10; (close reverse grip) 140 lb × 10, 140 lb × 8, 95 lb × 10

Dumbbell rows 40 lb × 12, 40 lb × 12, 45 lb × 10, 50 lb × 10, 50 lb × 10

Military press (machine) 60 lb × 15, 70 lb × 15, 80 lb × 15, 90 lb × 10, 60 lb × 8

Knee raises × 25, 25, 25, 25

SEBASTIAN STAN—MAY 20, 2013

Angie:

100 pull-ups

100 push-ups

100 sit-ups

100 squats

Total time 22:20.6

EXPERT TIP

How many times have you seen some dude in the gym doing seven different kinds of biceps exercises and just cruising through a workout? If you have to do that many curls to get through a workout, you are not expending enough energy doing one set. If I have you do barbell curls and we're going to do dumbbell curls afterward, you should look at me like I am the worst human on earth. You should have given me so much effort on those barbell curls that you should have nothing else to give. I don't like to see somebody at the gym doing four or five different kinds of biceps exercises. That's for body building professionals only. Be smart about what you are doing.

CHRIS PRATT—APRIL 29, 1013

Fight Gone Bad

Wall ball shots (20 lb ball) × 26, 18, 20, 16, 16

SDLHP (sumo dead lift high pulls) 75 lb × 17, 13, 15, 9, 9

Box jump (20-inch box) 13, 12, 12, 10, 13

Push presses 75 lb × 20, 25, 17, 12, 10

Row (kcal) × 13, 11, 10, 9, 13

Total score 379

ANNE HATHAWAY—AUGUST 20, 2013

Treadmill .5 mile easy: 8:12

Assisted pull-ups 80 lb × 10, 10, 10, 10

Assisted dips 80 lb × 10, 10, 10, 10

Squats × 10, 10, 10, 10

Sit-ups × 20, 20, 20, 20

Pulldowns 65 lb × 12, 70 lb × 10

TOM HIDDLESTON—MAY 23, 2011

Run 400 meters, 400 meters, 400 meters, 400 meters

Pull-ups × 10, 8, 6, 4

Push-ups × 20, 20, 20, 15

Glute Ham Developer (GHD) × 20, 20, 15, 12

Squats × 20, 20, 15, 15

Triceps extensions 50 lb × 12, 12, 10, 10

Dumbbell curls 25 lb × 15, 12, 10, 10

Burpees × 10, 10, 10, 10

Ball twist 10 lb ball × 20, 20, 15, 15

Row 400 meters, 440 meters, 400 meters, 400 meters

Total time 52:22.5

CHRIS PRATT—NOVEMBER 10, 2016

Treadmill warm-up 10 minutes easy

Dead lifts 135 × 15, 185 lb × 12, 205 lb × 12, 225 lb × 8, 245 lb × 6, 245 lb × 5

Hang cleans 45 lb × 12, 65 lb × 12, 95 lb × 10, 115 × 10

Shoulder press (machine) 80 lb × 15, 100 lb × 15, 110 lb × 12, 120 lb × 12, 120 lb × 12

Side cable lateral raises 20 lb × 12, 20 lb × 12, 20 lb × 12, 20 lb × 12

Ab machine 70 lb × 25, 25, 25, 25

JONAH HILL—MAY 4, 2017

Pull-ups × 5

Squats 45 lb × 15, 75 lb × 10, 100 lb × 10, 130 lb × 10, 150 lb × 6, 170 lb × 4, 190 lb × 1

Overhead presses 45 lb × 10, 75 lb × 8, 95 lb × 3, 110 lb × 1

Dead lifts 135 lb × 8, 165 lb × 4, 195 lb × 2, 215 lb × 1, 225 lb × 1

Bench press bar × 15, 95 lb × 10, 115 lb × 8, 135 lb × 6, 155 lb × 3, 175 lb × 1

Pulldowns 95 lb × 10, 110 lb × 8, 125 lb × 4, 140 lb × 3, 155 lb × 2, 170 lb × 1

PIERCE BROSNAN—MARCH 9, 2016

Chest presses 50 lb × 15, 70 lb × 15, × 15, × 10

Pulldowns 110 × 15, 12, 13, 12

Pec dec 30 lb × 15, 15, 15

Leg press 110 lb × 15, 140 lb × 15, 15, 15

Seated cable rows 65 lb × 15, 80 lb × 15, 15, 12

Air squats × 15, 15, 15, 15

Shoulder presses 30 lb × 15, 15, 15, 12

Superset

Leg extensions 40 lb × 15, 45 lb × 15, 15, 12

Leg curls 40 lb × 15, 15, 15, 15

Cable curls 30 lb × 15, 15, 15, 15

Standing triceps extensions 40 lb × 15, 45 lb × 15, 15, 15

Ab machine 60 lb × 50, 70 lb × 50, 80 lb × 50

AUGUSTO AGUILERA—OCTOBER 30, 2017

Row 1,000 meters easy: 4:18

Pull-ups × 5, push-ups × 10, squats × 15

Superset

Dumbbell rows 60 lb × 12, 70 lb × 10, 80 lb × 8, 8, 8, 8, 8, 8, 8, 8

Dumbbell bench presses 40 lb × 12, 50 lb × 10, 55 lb × 8, 8, 8, 8, 8, 8, 8, 8

MetCon

Pull-ups × 5, 5, 5, 5, 5, 5

Push-ups × 10, 10, 10, 10, 10, 10

Squats × 15, 15, 15, 15, 15, 15

Sit-ups × 20, 20, 20, 20, 20, 20

ADAM SANDLER—MAY 5, 2010

5 rounds of:

Run 400 meters, 400 meters, 400 meters, 400 meters,
400 meters

Pull-ups × 12, 12, 12, 12, 12

Push-ups × 20, 20, 20, 20, 20

Sit-ups × 20, 20, 20, 20, 20

Squats × 20, 20, 20, 20, 20

Assisted dips 60 lb × 12, 12, 12, 12, 12

EZ bar curls 60 lb × 12, 12, 12, 12, 12

Standing triceps extensions 100 lb × 12, 12, 12, 12, 12

Total time 44:40.76

ADAM SANDLER—MAY 8, 2010

3 10-minute AMRAPs

Pull-ups × 5 / push-ups × 10 / squats × 15 = 8 rounds

Burpees × 5 / dumbbell swings 30 × 10 / crunches × 15 = 6 rounds

Thrusters 20 lb × 10 / side crunch × 10 / dumbbell curls 20 lb × 10 = 6 rounds

SEBASTIAN STAN—MARCH 26, 2013

Warm-up: pull-ups × 15, push-ups × 20, squats × 25, sit-ups × 30, bridge 1 minute, sit-ups × 25, bridge 1 minute, sit-ups × 20, bridge 1 minute

Pulldowns 140 lb × 15, 155 lb × 12, 170 lb × 12, 185 lb × 10, 200 lb × 10, 215 lb × 7

Dumbbell rows 80 lb × 15, 80 lb 12, 12, 12, 12

Lying triceps extension 60 lb × 15, 70 lb × 12, 12, 10, 10

Standing triceps extension 65 lb × 15, 12, 12, 12

SCARLETT JOHANSSON—JULY 20, 2010

4 rounds of

Run 400 meters, 400 meters, 400 meters, 400 meters

Pull-ups × 12, 12, 12, 12

Push-ups × 12, 12, 12, 12

Glute Ham Developer (GHD) × 12, 12, 12, 12

Squats × 25, 25, 25, 25

Standing triceps extension 30 lb × 12, 12, 12, 12

Dumbbell curls 10 lb × 12, 12, 12, 12

Jump squats × 12, × 12, 12, 12

Ball twists 20 lb × 12, 12, 12, 12

Row 500 meters, 500 meters, 400 meters, 400 meters

Treadmill 10 min easy

Superset

Pulldowns 55 lb × 15, 15, 15, 15

Squats × 20, × 20, 20, 20

Dumbbell rows 15 lb × 15, 25 lb × 12, 12, 10

Push-ups (full) × 12, 12, 12, 12

Row 400 meters

Abs (crunches × 25; ball twists 10 × 25; side crunches × 25/25) × 4

Row 400 meters

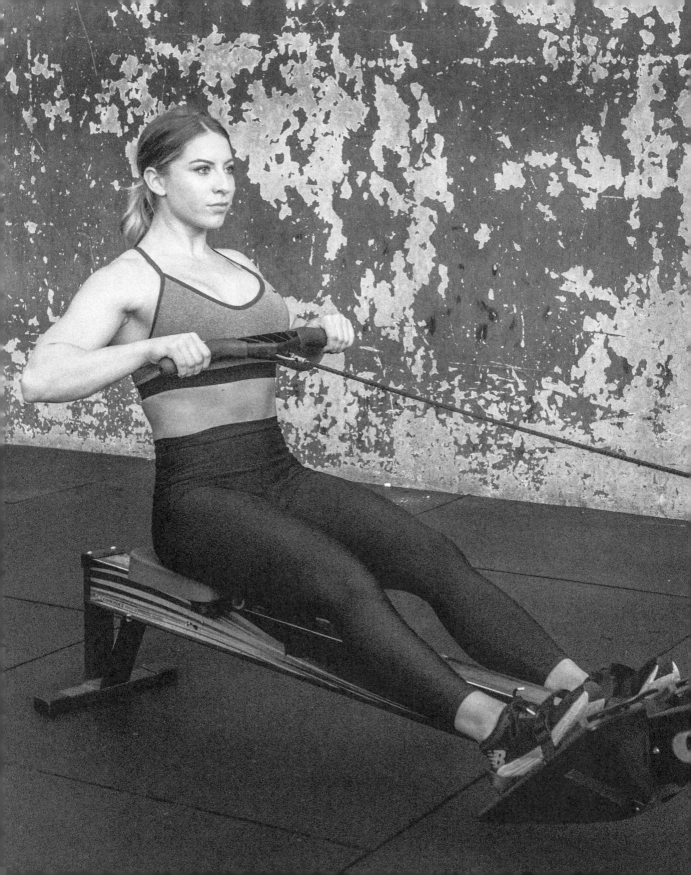

7

Cardio and Conditioning

Nobody else can take you to the place you want
to end up. You have to get there yourself.
—Tia-Clair Toomey, three-time Fittest Woman on Earth

What is the purpose of cardio? From a fitness standpoint, it's to get fat off the body. From a wellness
standpoint, you are training your body to get more
oxygen into your muscles. What do you want? You
want a strong pump house—your heart. So if overweight people are totally out of shape, they have poor conditioning. They need to care for all
this extra tissue. The body needs to be fed all this extra blood and oxygen.
Every time an overweight person does something physical, he or she has
to pause because the heart is working like a monster trying to supply
blood to all of this real estate. So we've got to bring the property size
down. We have to condition the heart to be more efficient to get blood/
oxygen out to the body, and at the same time we have to get the excess
body fat gone so that we have less real estate to tend.

The overweight person's heart is beating hard while he or she reads
a book or watches a movie, whereas a lean athlete's heart is on vacation.
As an overweight guy starts working out, he starts upping the workload,
conditioning his heart, putting big oxygen demands on his body. As he
loses weight, his pump gets stronger, his arteries get enlarged and cleaned

out, and then his body gets more efficient. As you get fitter, now it's about trying to work in an oxygen deficit. We're walking along and you and I are talking. We're not working hard. So let's start walking faster, move into an easy jog. Two guys out for a jog. Now we pick up our pace at the park. You are breathing hard. Your body is trying to get oxygen to accomplish the work you want to do; it needs you to shut up so you can do the work. Now we pick up the work a little more. I ask, "How are the wife and kids?" All you can say is "Great!" You don't want to talk anymore because you are at the top of your aerobic capacity. You're getting in all the oxygen you need to accomplish the demand on your body. At a certain point, your body can't take in enough oxygen to do the work. That point is where glucose gets burned up, where the fatty tissue you are still trying to get rid of also goes.

So why am I telling you all of this? Because I want you to know that there are different ways to do cardio. Each way has a different purpose, so you have to tailor the cardio or conditioning you are doing to what you are trying to accomplish. A person who is already really lean and needs to be quick doesn't need to be doing a lot of steady-state cardio (unless they want to be an endurance athlete), while a person who is very overweight needs to get rid of a lot of that excess weight. It all works. I just want folks to understand what one program does as opposed to another.

DON'T MAKE IT COMPLICATED. KEEP IT SIMPLE.

I'll be the first to admit high-intensity interval training (HIIT) is not for everyone. It has become very popular in the last few years. It's still useful, and I'm not going to say don't do it. But the old-school stuff still works, and for most people, that's probably what you are going to want to do. HIIT is hard, and often it is used to improve performance in a specific sport. Yes, it is very effective. But you do end up tiring yourself out more and it can increase the chance for injury. What's gotten a bad rap these days is good old-fashioned steady-state cardio. It's the easiest approach to losing weight and the safest to improving heart health.

Jogging has always been the most effective weight-loss regimen there is. But I'll also be first one to tell you that you need to do more than just jog, because the motion of picking your foot up and putting it down is not a natural range of motion and will hurt you as you age. You can also use a rowing machine or any piece of cardio equipment that will get your heart rate up to a high enough level that you are entering the fat-burning zone.

Unfortunately stationary bikes and elliptical machines, while great tools, are not very effective at elevating your heart rate into this zone. So unless you are injured or elderly, I would not recommend using one of those machines. The amount of effort required to elevate the heart rate is just too difficult to sustain over a period of time. Something that works your total body is better.

The fat-burning zone is the target heart rate that optimizes your ability to burn fat. You'll find a formula online you can follow. But I have always tried to make things simple by using 180 minus your age as a rule of thumb. That gets you to about where your heart rate should be to burn fat. Ten points lower than that also works. Anything above or below is not where you want to be. If you go too high, you stop burning fat as your source of energy and start tapping into glucose and glycogen. And if you go too low, you aren't working hard enough to burn all that much fat, so you're not going to see a lot of change.

Let me make sure that this advice is clear. For example, you see an overweight woman or man in a spin class just huffing and puffing, soaring past all of their aerobic stuff. They are not burning fat. What they are burning out of their system is glucose and glycogen, meaning that they are just burning calories. When she or he is done, there's a greater chance that they are going to eat a lot afterward to replace everything that they've lost. They will get fatter because they are not paying attention to their goals or their heart rate. You can spin your spin, do your class, but if

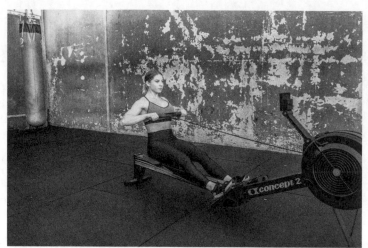

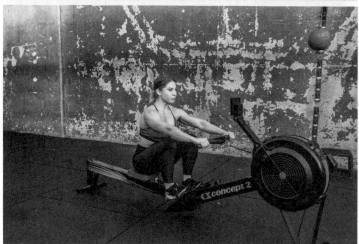

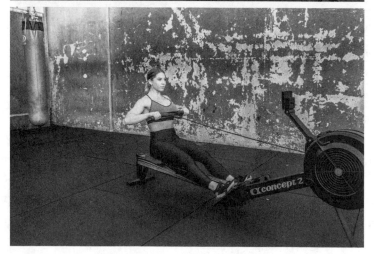

you are there for fat loss, you need to be in that window I just gave you. To pinpoint that range effectively, you need to use a heart rate monitor. It's the easiest, simplest way to burn fat effectively.

If you don't have a heart rate monitor, you can also check your perceived exertion, a way of measuring the intensity of your physical activity. You want to be doing cardio at a pace such that if you were jogging and talking to someone, you couldn't speak in complete sentences. You should be able to speak, but only in short words. That's the pace you should be traveling at.

Steady-state cardio carries with it a minimum chance of injury, and it increases your cardio output, which makes you a better lifter and overall improves your endurance. This in turn greatly improves your overall health—namely your heart health.

It has worked for centuries. I'm a big fan of it. It still works. Why change it?

EXPERT TIP: WHAT NOT TO DO

A while back I was going for runs on a track in Los Angeles and training for triathlons. I still remember passing three women decked out in their fancy workout clothes. Energy drinks clipped to their waists, they were walking slowly on the track, just chatting it up while the other runners were training hard. That's not fitness. That's social hour. Leave that at the café. You want to go out and exercise, then exercise. Stop coming up with half-baked notions of how you can make exercising more pleasant. It requires real effort and your full attention. What you put into it is often what you get out of it.

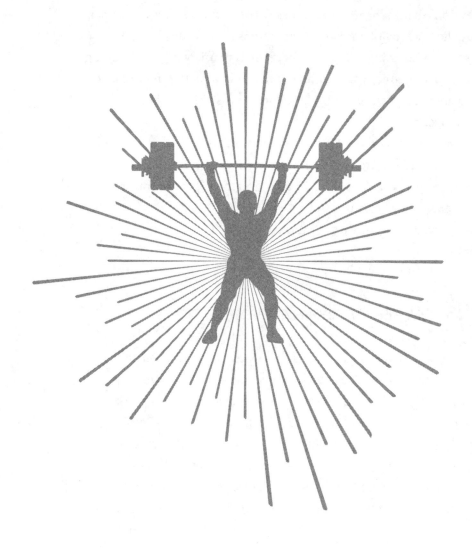

SAMPLE CARDIO PROGRESSION

WEEK 1

Monday—30 minutes

Tuesday—30 minutes

Wednesday—30 minutes

Thursday—30 minutes

Friday—30 minutes

Saturday—30 minutes

Sunday—rest

WEEK 2

Monday—35 minutes

Tuesday—35 minutes

Wednesday—35 minutes

Thursday—35 minutes

Friday—35 minutes

Saturday—35 minutes

Sunday—rest

WEEK 3

Monday—40 minutes

Tuesday—40 minutes

Wednesday—40 minutes

Thursday—40 minutes

Friday—40 minutes

Saturday—40 minutes

Sunday—rest

WEEK 4

Monday—45 minutes

Tuesday—45 minutes

Wednesday—45 minutes

Thursday—45 minutes

Friday—45 minutes

Saturday—45 minutes

Sunday—rest

WEEK 5

Monday—50 minutes

Tuesday—50 minutes

Wednesday—50 minutes

Thursday—50 minutes

Friday—50 minutes

Saturday—50 minutes

Sunday—rest

Once you've comfortably made it to 50 minutes, you can back off or continue at 50 minutes, depending on where you are. Once in a while you're going to want to reset to get yourself going again.

And make sure you show signs of progression so that you keep moving forward.

CONDITIONING OPTIONS

I work in the film business, and my clients have different needs. Not everyone who comes to me needs to do a lot of cardio. Sometimes my clients are already lean and just need to be ripped and focus on speed work. Whatever they may need, at the end of the day, I am responsible for making people look good or giving the actor or studio the look that they want. So that's predominantly where my focus lies. That said, there are other options out there besides traditional cardio. If you are a lean person looking to do something different or if steady-state cardio is not your cup of tea, then here are some options for you to explore. Just understand: Whatever you focus on, there are upsides and downsides to each option. For example, if you do HIIT exclusively and all of a sudden you want to run a marathon, you are going to struggle.

You need to determine what it is you are trying to accomplish in order to find the program that works best for you.

JUMPING ROPE

This is still one of the most effective ways to exercise your heart and your legs. If you are capable of skipping rope for 20 to 30 minutes at a time and you enjoy it, go for it.

HIIT

Here are two sample HIIT workouts:

1. Sprint up a hill 20 times, using 85 to 100 percent max effort. Rest about 2 minutes between the sprints, usually while you are walking back down the hill.
2. If you don't have a hill, use a treadmill set at an incline and follow the same procedure.

A VARIATION ON CROSSFIT CINDY

Complete as many rounds in 20 minutes as you can. Keep track of how many times you get through it and chart your progress.

5 pull-ups

10 push-ups

15 sit-ups

20 air squats

KETTLEBELLS

Here are two very effective kettlebell workouts that will leave you gasping for air. Try to do this with as little rest as possible.

10 kettlebell swings; 10 burpees

9 kettlebell swings; 9 burpees

8 kettlebell swings; 8 burpees

Etc.

All the way down till you get to zero.

Four or five rounds of:

10 kettlebell swings

10 lunges

10 presses

10 squats

10 Turkish gets-ups*

Rest 2 minutes between rounds, or only 1 if you want more of a challenge.

HEAVY CARRIES AND PUSHES

One of the most terrific ways to improve endurance and burn fat is to do heavy carries or pushes. This isn't for everyone, and you need space to do this. But a carry simply involves just picking up something heavy and walking with it, whether that's a farmer's carry involving two dumbbells, a medicine ball, a single heavy kettlebell, or buckets filled with water, it doesn't matter.

If you happen to be lucky and have access to a sled, training with such equipment can also be a great way to improve your work capacity. At a minimum you want to load a sled up with the equivalent of your body weight and push it around or pull it. This can be a great way to finish a workout.

CONCLUSION

Do what works best for your goals. Go at the pace that you need to. So, for example, if you can't run for 30 minutes at a stretch, don't despair. Just go run around the block and then walk the rest of the time and keep trying to improve each time you go for a run. You just have to put in the effort. Just ask your body and your body will step up. If you are in a wheelchair or have an injury that keeps you from running, then go swim.

---

* Check out the video for how to perform the Turkish get-up on YouTube: https://www.youtube.com/watch?v=-_zTytmHM94.

Swim half a lap the first time. Swim three-quarters of a lap the next time. If you can run a 7-minute mile, great. The next time you go out, run 6:55. The whole thing here is progressive training. You need to keep improving, and if you aren't, then you need to change something.

TIPS

- Use a heart rate monitor to keep yourself in the fat-burning zone.
- Make sure you pay attention to form.
- Make sure you don't rely on one thing too much. Too much endurance will make you lose HIIT ability and too much HIIT will result in poor endurance; you want to be balanced.
- If you are really looking to bulk up, go easy on the cardio

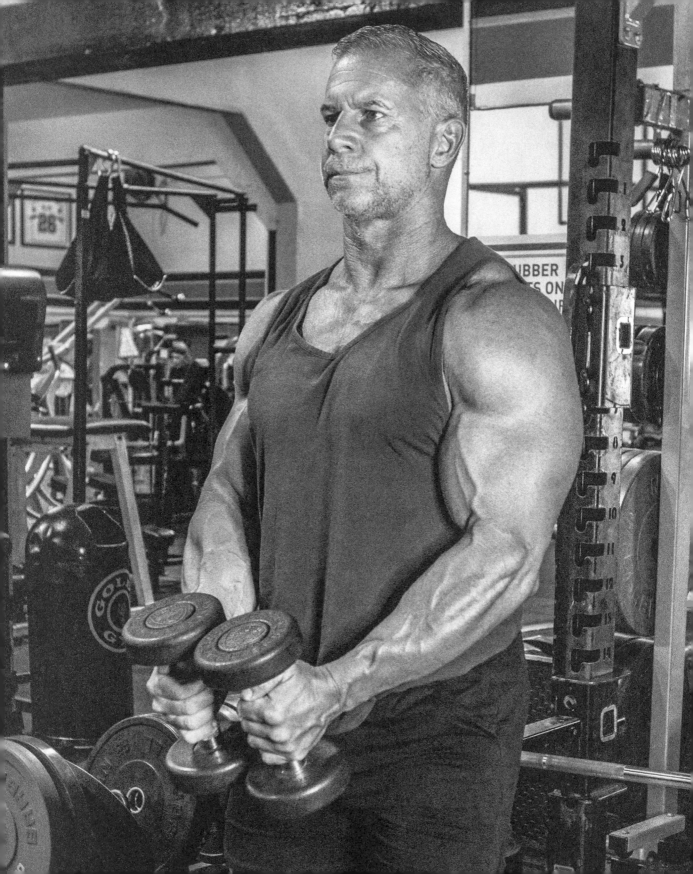

Nutrition

Fruit-wise when I competed, I'd have 12 blueberries with my
oatmeal every other morning. And on low carb days, 3 ounces
of pineapple with my two beef meals that day.
—Richard "Flex" Lewis, trainer and body builder

GETTING YOUR EATING RIGHT

People might think this is the hardest thing for them to wrap
their heads around. But it's not hard. Everyone says they
don't know how to eat. I'll bet that you do but you just
don't realize it. Again, as with all the other things I've talked
about, it's not complicated. The industry has made it complicated. So
let's *un*complicate it.

Okay, I'm going to give you two plates. There's a pile of doughnuts on
one plate and two chicken breasts on the other. Which one do you eat?

If you picked chicken—great. You're a nutritionist.

That's the first step.

You know the difference between good food and bad food. You've
known it since you were a little kid. Your mother knows it, your grandma
knows it. But everything is about the choices you make. If you're eating well, then the next discussion is about how much food should be on
the plate. I put in front of you a pile of salad and a generous portion of

chicken breast. On the other plate is a pile of chicken breasts and a side of salad. Which do you eat?

If you're eating the single chicken breast with the salad, you're now a genius nutritionist.

It's not hard once you stop to think about it. The hard part is making the right choices. And you already know what they are. Rarely do you run into a kind of food where you don't know if it's good for you or not. Big businesses, like the food industry, have programmed us to think differently. Well, don't think differently. Stick to what you know, to what you learned a long time ago. Healthy eating comes in the form of eating whole foods. The more whole foods you eat, the healthier and leaner you are going to be.

This is not rocket science. Don't make it complicated. Every bit of what you eat is stored up as energy. If you're taking in more calories than you need, you're proceeding in the wrong direction. Doesn't matter what you're eating or how much exercise you are getting.

STUFF YOU SHOULD EAT OFTEN

Lean red meats, skinless chicken, pork, skinless turkey, lean burger meat or turkey burger, lean chicken, lamb

Fish

Salmon or tuna fillets, lobster, trout, shrimp, mahimahi, wild tuna and salmon in a pouch or can

Eggs—organic, 100 percent free range

Vegetables—organic and fresh (preferably dark leafy greens or cruciferous vegetables)

Asparagus, bell peppers, lettuce, cabbage, broccoli, zucchini, leeks, kale, green beans, spinach

STUFF TO EAT IN MODERATION

Most fruit, starchy vegetables, nuts, seeds

STUFF NOT TO EAT

Why would you need this list? You're trying to get into the best shape of your life.

SAMPLE MENU

DAY 1

Breakfast
Eggs
Brown rice
Broccoli

Midday snack
Turkey
Avocado slices

Lunch
Grilled salmon
Asparagus

Midday snack
Almonds

Dinner

Lean steak

Brussels sprouts

DAY 2

Breakfast

Eggs

Oatmeal

Spinach

Small chicken breast

Midday snack

Chicken

Broccoli

Brown rice

Lunch

Grilled steak

Asparagus

Brown rice

Midday snack

Apple

Turkey meat

Dinner

Grilled lemon chicken

Legumes

DAY 3

Breakfast

Eggs

Brown rice

Broccoli

Midday snack

Beef jerky (low sodium)

Lunch

Grilled salmon

Asparagus

Midday snack

Almonds

Dinner

Lean steak

Brussels sprouts

I think you get the idea.

You can mix up the foods, but you are sticking to the same game plan of eating the healthiest foods you can find—the leanest pieces of meat, dark leafy greens, brown rice, or oatmeal—to get a little energy in you.

Someone came up with a great saying about nutrition: eat like a king for breakfast, a prince for lunch, and a pauper for dinner. I've always liked that proverb. Just think about it. When you wake up, you need energy, and as you go through your day, you need energy, but you don't need energy just before you go to sleep. In fact your food will digest better if your evening meal is the lightest one. You should be about 75 to 80 percent full at that point of the day.

> ## EXPERT TIP: AVOIDING CRAVINGS
>
> Say you are feeling shitty. What do you do? You're home and you go to your refrigerator and you start finding food. Why? Because if you can stuff shit in your mouth, you will feel better than you felt a minute before, so that's what you're looking for. *Don't. Don't walk toward the kitchen. Walk outside. Head for the gym. Do something. Walk to the store and buy a bottle of water. Don't walk there for chocolate doughnuts. Walk in the direction of shit that's on your side.*

CUT OUT THE JUNK

Most people understand that you can't suck down double cheeseburgers and fries to get fit. But you also don't need all the junk the fitness industry peddles at you. Protein bars, for example, are a waste of your money. I like to call them get-you-fat bars. They will make you fat and will keep you from getting lean. They're full of junk, and they're a huge part of the industry. So are the powders. They have powders for everything—workout powders, protein powders, pump powders, mental focus powders, you name it. The labels don't mean the powders do anything. Cut out the junk. What about thermogenic supplements? No. When you eat a piece of food and you feel full, your body is going to work on breaking that food down. That's thermogenesis. You don't need something to help it along. Your body already does it. Use your body correctly. You can't cheat your way to fitness.

Not long ago, I was at the gym and saw this giant guy in the parking lot. He had enormous arms and legs and was jacked beyond belief, and he also had a huge gut. He had the trunk of his car open, and in there was just about every type of powder and artificial drink mix you could possibly get your hands on. All I could think was *Dude, I wish you had a trainer. Throw all of that garbage out. Eat a good diet. Mix it up. Stop doing all the crazy lifting and get yourself ripped.* If he dropped ten pounds, he would have looked phenomenal, the way most of us dream about.

Make smart decisions. Don't be a dumb-ass.

EXPERT TIP: TRY THIS CHALLENGE

If you can spend six days eating like this, then you can do anything. Oatmeal, eggs, and spinach for breakfast. Chicken, broccoli, and brown rice for lunch, chicken, broccoli, brown rice for a snack, then chicken and broccoli for dinner. Do this for six days and you will be amazed at how different you look and feel. When you complete that challenge, then you can start substituting different proteins and carbohydrates.

CARBOHYDRATES

Carbohydrates are not bad. You need them for energy and putting on size. Your age, your size, and your goals for yourself determine the number of carbohydrates you need. You definitely need carbs around the time you work out. But later in the day, unless you are trying to get huge, you don't. If you are trying to get ripped, I would limit them. If you are overweight, I would limit them to the point that you lose the weight and then reintroduce around the time you are exercising. You want to be eating complex carbohydrates. So focus on foods like sweet potatoes, brown rice, oatmeal, and so forth.

CHEAT MEAL

What's a cheat meal? I think you probably know. It's that one meal you are allowed to eat one day a week in order to stay sane: pizza, a bagel, pasta, fried wings, ice cream. Cheat meals are not an all-you-can-eat buffet. We're talking about one meal once during the week, not an entire day of cheating. And you don't get cheat meals until you have your diet under control, because then what's the point? So if you are nailing your diet, have a cheat meal. If you aren't, then wait until you've gotten yourself under control.

OTHER DIETS

The ketogenic diet has become very popular lately. So has intermittent fasting. Keto works. Chicken, broccoli, and brown rice totally works, too. All the programs you see people touting work. If you put 100 percent of your effort into keto, it will work. If you go chicken, broccoli, and brown rice 100 percent, it works. If you generally eat right most of the time, it works. If you eat right in a half-ass manner, forget it. Remember will, desire, and discipline. Apply that to any method of healthy eating that you want, and it works. However, if you are going to give only 75 percent in these programs, then you are going to get 75 percent results. All this stuff works only if you apply yourself 100 percent.

All of it is just 100 percent distraction if you half-ass it. So don't half-ass it.

If you have 100 percent focus, then it's all about picking the one that is going to work for you.

EXPERT TIP

For the period during which you're really trying to make progress, you don't need fruit; if you do want to incorporate it into your day, eat it early, eat small quantities of it, and eat it on your cheat day.

WHAT YOU SHOULD DRINK

Water is what you are supposed to drink. You're made out of it. So here's the plan: drink water.

Look at the animal. This is what your body needs. If you don't drink water, you can feel how screwed up your body gets.

If you don't drink milk or soda, you survive.

If you stop drinking water, eventually you die.

You also need to drink a *lot* of water, more than you are probably drinking right now. The average person doesn't hydrate enough, and water has a ton of benefits, not least of which is it helps you lean out. It helps you flush out the body. It promotes thermogenesis and a feeling of fullness, and it enhances the body's performance.

How much of it should you be drinking? Here's a formula you can use if you want, or you can just DRINK.

Multiply your weight by 2/3 to calculate how much water you need to drink on a daily basis. For example, if you weigh 160 pounds, the calculation will be as follows: $160 \times 2/3 = 107$ ounces (3.16 liters) of water per day.

Or simply look at your urine when you go to the bathroom. If it's dark yellow, you're not drinking enough. If it's clear, then you are doing a good job.

SUPPLEMENTS

There are a billion supplements out there. People want to use creatine or protein power or thermogenic supplements. Let me emphasize this. What's your reason for using any of this stuff? You don't need it. So many people got so fit without it. Some of it isn't totally useless. But let's not get sidetracked. Are such supplements necessary for you to achieve the goals you have in mind? The answer is no. Save your money.

What riles me up the most about supplements is that they all use what's known as a "proprietary blend." You'll see those words on almost every training-related product. *Proprietary blend* means that manufacturers will put in whatever the hell they feel like. As is true with, say, cocaine, the active ingredient is expensive, but the filler is cheap. The more filler manufacturers pack in your supplement, the better it is for them. Thus the fitness supplement industry mirrors the drug trade.

TIPS

- If you have to go out to eat, ask them to prepare something exactly the way you want it or have a small snack beforehand to help fill you up.
- Every time you feel hungry, drink water.
- Your focus on eating should be on par with the focus you bring to the gym.

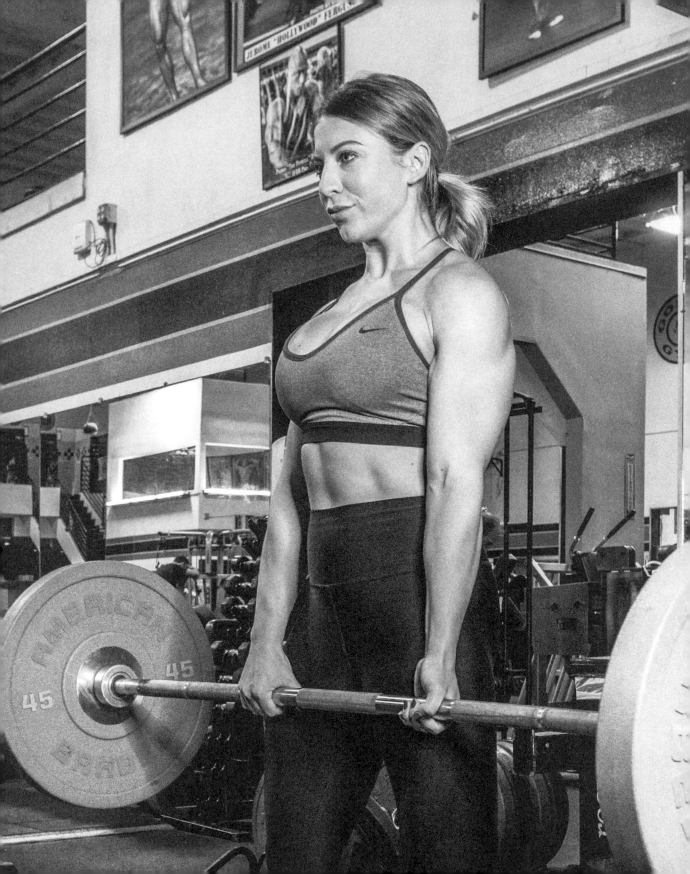

Recovery

Be humble, be hungry, and always be the hardest worker in the room.
—Dwayne "The Rock" Johnson

When you are working your body really hard, you must do the things you need to do to keep your body and your mental focus at a high level. To be a SEAL, you wake up every day and work out hard until your lungs feel like they're bleeding and your muscles feel like they are going to snap. Then when the day is over, you need food and sleep, and as much of these as you can get. That's the kind of recovery you get in the SEALs. You're taking your body to the highest levels of human performance. If you are starring in a movie with a $250 million budget, you need to be in as good a shape as you've ever been in your life. You are training with maximal effort, so you need to eat with precision and get enough sleep. You're getting the crap kicked out of you at the gym, lifting weights, doing cardio, stunt training, etc. So you need to recover as best you can every day.

Some of you reading this might think, *Okay, that makes sense. But how can I do what an actor or actress does when they have an entire support system to hold them up?* By this, I mean they might be able to take an ice bath or the studio will pay for a deep tissue massage. Does that stuff help? Sure, in some small way. But SEALs don't have any of that and they still reach amazing levels of fitness. Don't let anything stand in your way. Such things don't make or break you. If you forget to have a protein shake or you can't afford one, so long as you're eating right, your muscles will recover. The decision that you are going to get fit matters far more than whether you get a massage or if you have an instructor screaming at you or a trainer talking to you at the gym. You can have a company deliver meals with the exact nutrients you need or you can go to Costco and cook all your meals in bulk and freeze single-size portions. You can have someone make you a smoothie or you can have what you need in your kitchen and bang one out before you go to work.

The most important parts of recovery have nothing to do with deep tissue massage for your muscles or drinking a protein shake immediately after you work out. Eating right is hugely effective. Nutritious foods help you grow stronger and recover. They provide the proper vitamins and minerals and energy to keep your body performing.

Getting the proper amount of rest will also improve your performance. Sleep is hugely important in the building of muscle. You need a good seven to eight hours of sleep a night if you want to build muscle effectively and lose fat. There's no way around this. (And by the way, spending money on Tom Brady's recovery pajamas isn't going to get you there. I'm sure they're nice, but they have zero bearing on your success.) The fact is, your body needs rest; *you* need rest. It is essential to your body's ability to function. Strenuous physical activity puts stress on your muscles and your nervous system. These are rebuilt during sleep. Your pituitary gland releases growth hormones, which help your muscle tissues heal.

How do you get good sleep? That's in your camp. You've got to set up an environment that allows you to get adequate rest. And look, we all have constraints in our daily lives—jobs, long commutes, caring for our kids, anything that gets in the way. But at the end of the day, you need to take care of yourself. What good are you if you are not rested? If you are going to put your body through strenuous physical activity, let your body heal so that you can keep going.

Actors have arduous schedules and can find it hard to get the sleep they need. They might have to be up early for a shoot or table read. So what I tell my clients is, if you can't get the full eight hours you need, take naps. Stop what you are doing when you have a moment and take a short nap. Get as much rest as you can.

And again, you need proper hydration. If you aren't drinking enough water, you aren't flushing all the toxins out of your body and keeping your machine running at peak efficiency.

STRETCHING AND FOAM ROLLERS

People often ask about stretching. I have an easy answer to that question, one that probably surprises people. You can't get more stretched out than when you are doing your exercises properly. If you are going deep into a squat, that's a stretch. If you are taking that bench press bar to your chest and all the way out, you're stretching. If you are doing pulls-ups from a dead hang, you're getting in a good stretch. The same goes for a military press. If you are getting that bar all the way up and then down, good. You are stretching. The reason I don't feel the need to emphasize stretching with my clients is that there are enough distractions as it is, and if you are exercising correctly and taking care of yourself, this stuff is less important. If you like doing it, go for it. I'm not going to tell you no. Just don't let it get in the way of the things you *have* to do. I don't want people distracted by this stuff. It's just another thing for you to worry about when you don't need to.

The same goes for foam rollers. I know people love them. There are foam rollers that vibrate and ones with deep grooves in them; these are supposedly helpful. But look, people did just fine before any of this stuff came along. It's just a product, a product that made some company a lot of money.

All I can tell you definitively (and I've said this once before) is that warming up is important, and it becomes far more important as you age. And if you are going to stretch, stretch *after* you warm up, not before. You need your muscles to be warm. Warm muscles prevent injury.

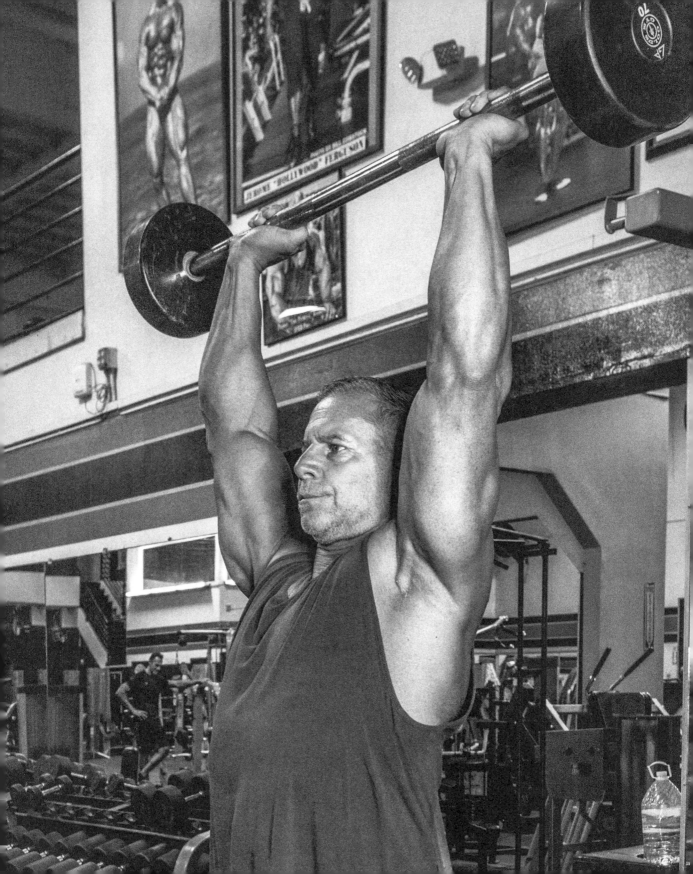

10

Closing Thoughts

Training gives us an outlet for suppressed energies created by stress and thus tones the spirit just as exercise conditions the body.
—Arnold Schwarzenegger

MILO OF CROTON

There's a lot to be learned from the Greeks, and the story of Milo of Croton is a perfect example of what fitness is. Some 2,500 years ago, Milo of Croton, a man renowned for his incredible strength and athleticism, was the most successful wrestler of his day, a six-time champion at the Olympic games in Greece. The legends of his strength and training have been told time and again. He's a figure often used to demonstrate the principles of fitness. As the story goes, a newborn calf was born near Milo's home, so the wrestler decided to lift the small animal and carry him on his shoulders. Milo did this every day for 4 years until he was carrying a full-size bull upon his shoulders.

This is an early story of progressive resistance. It's the story of a man who was determined to grow stronger and did it by progressively overloading his body until he was fit enough to handle the demands of a growing workload. And of a man who was determined to improve, knowing that the massive changes he was looking for would come about only over time.

This is what fitness is. It's having the will, the discipline, and the desire to succeed. Milo knew what he was doing, and he became the strongest guy in town by implementing it. With very little equipment and a lot of will, he forged himself into a champion. This simple story contains a great lesson, so keep it in mind as you approach your training and your diet. Try to get yourself going in the direction you want to be going in.

DISTRACTIONS

Life is full of distractions, especially in today's media-driven world, so it's important to zero in on what matters. When it comes to getting fit, what matters is a total focus on what you are doing—nothing else. Let's take music, for example. We all love to listen to music, particularly when we exercise. Some gyms even blast it. If your music selection is distracting you, turning you into a deejay or making you go all John Travolta and dance, just generally slowing you down, then get rid of it. Back in the day I used earplugs while I did squats with a buddy of mine. All you can hear is your own breathing. It improves your focus and ratchets up your intensity.

The same goes for if you are watching TV at the gym or at home while you are exercising—stop doing it. There's no way you are working your hardest (and effectively using your limited time) when you are watching TV. In fact, if you are able to exercise while you are watching TV, I would say you aren't really working at all, you are half-assing it. Save that for an off day.

And your phone. Whoa! People can't do anything without cell phones these days. If you can't drive a car while using your phone, then you shouldn't be using your phone while you exercise. It's a *major* distraction. You are not going to give even close to 100 percent if you are playing with your phone. You're just not. There's no reason for you to be glued to it.

Checking your feed or reading your email is not going to improve your fitness, but it will hold you back.

Don't do any of this. Be smart. When you are engaged in getting fit, that's your time to get fit. All that other stuff is for later.

CHOOSING A GYM

Many people want to go to the best gym or to have the best trainer. Well, let's be honest, you can't always have the best. In fact the best isn't always the right gym for you. If the best gym is an hour away from your home and there's a perfectly fine gym five minutes away, don't go to the one that's an hour away; instead go to the one that's close to home. Odds are you will use it more often and will have more free time as a result. That's just the way it is. Also, your gym should make you feel welcome. If the atmosphere or the people at the gym make you feel uncomfortable, go to another gym. Or go to that gym and set a new tone for the culture. Get yourself in fantastic shape and help get other people fit. Don't hoard information. Share your knowledge. And if you're going to hire a trainer, make sure that person has your goals in mind. Make sure the trainer knows what he or she is doing—watching your form, monitoring your diet, all of that.

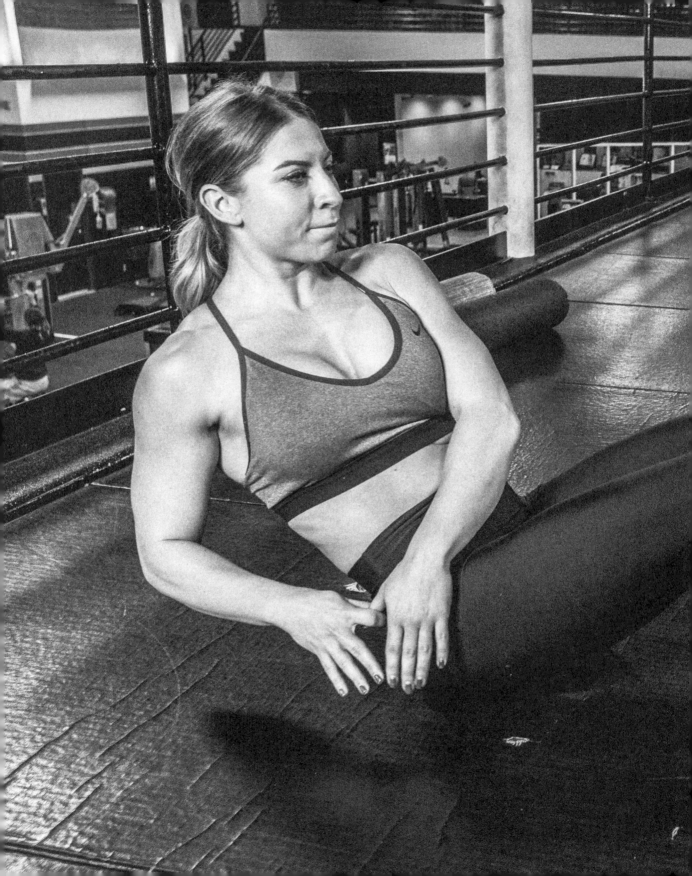

A Final Note

I hope whoever reads this book gets more fit as a result. I'm not concerned with your turning yourself into Chris Hemsworth. I'm concerned with your getting in better shape than you used to be. That's what it's all about: progression and improvement.

In this book I am addressing you in exactly the same way I have spoken with the A-listers who star in the movies you love. There are no hidden tricks. All the material I've included here is the same as what they get. It happens to be hands-on and not in a book, but it's all the knowledge I have. And they work for it, and you can work for it, too. There's nothing that they do that you can't do, too. We're all made up of the same tissues. Celebrities don't have a genetic advantage; if ordinary people put in the work, they can attain what stars do. Reaching the peak of your physical fitness is just about how much you want it and how hard you are going to work to get it. If you don't have a personal chef or meals being prepared for you by a service, so what? Body builders don't have that, and they look great. They're preparing all of their own meals and going on the road, and somehow they make it work. You can, too.

I have given you all the secrets. I have unmasked the fitness industry and the nonsense they propagate so that you can make more informed decisions about your health. Just as with everything else in these pages, you know everything you need to know. *You* are in charge. *You* are the one making the decisions on what to eat, carrying out the workouts, and then seeing to it that you get the proper rest.

I know it can be difficult. I know it's hard to fit fitness into your life sometimes, especially when it hasn't been a priority before. And there are challenges all around us. At the office, someone is always leaving out cake and cookies. It's so tempting, and other people do partake in the snacks, so why shouldn't you? You have to control those urges. Or maybe you're in a situation where you are married with kids and both you and your spouse are overweight. One of you wants to do something about it, and the other one doesn't. Well, that is a tough situation, but you've got to navigate it. Make your partner or whoever may make eating clean or exercising a little more challenging understand what it is that you want. The partner can always step up, too. There's no greater feeling than accomplishing your goals together and improving your health, holding each other accountable.

Health and fitness are supremely important to your life. At the end of the day your kids are going to grow up and leave home. All you are going to want at that point is your health. You're going to want both the health you used to have and the health you don't have. So maybe a little vanity helps you out in the long run. You are going to wish you had more time; you are going to wish you were healthier. As you age, your mind might start to go. Your mind works more clearly when you are physically healthy. Fitness can give you that. Studies have shown time and again the benefits of exercise for both body and mind—and no doctor is going to tell you *not* to exercise. You may be twenty years old right now and want to look like Thor, but I've got news for you—when you turn seventy, you are going to be glad you have fitness in your life. You will be a functioning person. You'll live a longer, fuller, and more joyful life as a result.

Keep something else in mind. If you ever want to set a good example for your kids, let them see you take care of your health. Show them that you care about yourself. It will do them a world of good. YOU are the superhero, in whatever form that takes—the mom of three who is still managing to get in her five A.M. morning run; the single dad who is staying fit at fifty; the couple who makes time to train together. Whatever you do, if you have kids, they watch you (they're *always* watching you), and if they see you busting your butt to take care of yourself, they will take care of themselves, too. Find inspiration in that. Another way to look at that is like this. How do you want your kids to see you? If they see you sitting on the couch being fat and tired, are you good with that? Do you want them to think you are lazy? If you go to Disney World with them and you're huffing and puffing up the stairs and they're running up, yelling "Come on!," do you think that's a good look for you? Nobody wants that. So do something about it. Stop being tired. Stop eating badly. Take control of your life.

Some of you may ask, "Well, what do I do if I'm making kid food and I need to stay on my healthy food track, but at the end of the day I'm too tired to cook after I get them food?" This is a huge concern for many people. But you have a few choices. You can make the kid food and then take care of your food, or you can try to make things easier for yourself by getting them to lean in your direction. So if you're eating a chicken breast and broccoli and they want to eat breaded fish sticks, make them the fish sticks and give them the broccoli, too. Let them see you making healthy choices and start encouraging them to have some healthy foods as well. I'm not saying it's going to be easy, but you have to be as focused about what you eat as you are about how you exercise and it's not such a terrible idea to try to keep your kids eating healthy, too. Pass good habits on to them. It's a struggle for sure, but wolfing down the pizza they are eating because you're tired is not the solution.

I've told you about the fitness industry. They need to make money. They're a business. Your health is *your* business, though. You need to look after it and you need to listen to what makes sense. Will, desire, discipline—they make sense. You can take those traits anywhere. They can transform your body and your health. When you go through BUD/S training, you will think of a hundred possible reasons to quit. If you want a reason to quit, you will find one. But if you are on the fence, then get on the fitness side of things, and if you already are on the fitness side of things, then ask for more. If you need a little bit of help, then get a personal trainer. There are great personal trainers out there. Do the necessary research and find a good one. And when you do find one, listen to them. You've hired a trainer for a reason. Trust them to do their job, which is making you fit. If they don't do that or they hurt you, find someone else.

You've got to work really hard. You've got to earn your reps. Chris Pratt persevered through his workouts until he transformed his whole body, and arguably his entire career along with it. Chris Hemsworth became mammoth and ripped. He put in the time. He's very dedicated. Scarlett Johansson kicked butt and got into the best shape of her life. You've got to reach for the stars to get bodies like that. That's what these A-listers do. True, they do need to get from point A to point B, but it's still on them, it's still the work they put into it.

EXPERT TIP: FINDING TIME

Q: Duff, what with the job, kids, and a family, I have trouble finding time to work out. What can I do?

A: Find the time. There are tons of distractions throughout your day. Get rid of the time wasters and find your time there. Get up early in the morning and go work out. If that doesn't work for you, what about lunchtime? If the middle of the day is bad, do you have time to do something in your office, or if you are traveling, can you use the hotel gym? You always have time. You just have to carve it out of your day.

While this exercise thing isn't for everyone, don't let anybody tell you that you can't do this stuff. And people will. A friend, a brother, a sister, a coworker, a stranger—somebody will give you a hard time about what you are trying to do. Just stay positive and look for the road that takes you forward.

There are many ways to be humbled by physical prowess. The gym is not one of those places. I still work as a stuntman occasionally, and when I'm on those sets, I see some of the greatest specialists galore at work. Some of these people perform such amazing feats of athleticism that it blows my mind just watching them. Get intimidated by seeing people do amazing things. Admire them. Don't get intimidated by someone pumping iron at the gym. That's stupid. They were you once.

So whether you do my programs or not, do something—anything. If you are trying to lose weight, don't talk to people about it; instead set down a goal and go for it. If you are trying to take your fitness to another level, set yourself up with the proper plan and follow through to accomplish that goal—you don't want to be stuck in a rut for years grinding out the same workout and going nowhere. Be smart, have faith, and you will find that path forward.

If you recall my analogy from the beginning of the book, there are three types of clients. There are the ones that get on the autobahn and go 100 miles an hour, and they eat great, train great, and sleep great. Then there are those who take the 405 and they do it all well, but they're not 100 percent in. Then there are those people who take the back roads and ride over potholes. They're not going to make it at all.

You don't know me. I don't know you. But I want you to succeed. Get a real look at yourself, understand what type of body you have, and focus on getting the best body that you can. Don't compare yourself to other people, especially people you will never look like. You might not get ripped in twelve weeks, and hey, that's okay. Really, it is. It can take months or years. Some people may never make it. But don't be the person that laments the doughnut he or she just ate and whines about it to others. Be the person who tries to do something about it. And if you don't want to do something about it, then don't complain about it. Stop coming up with excuses and live the healthiest, fullest life that you can. We're not here forever. But there are things you can control, there are changes you can make to your life and your lifestyle, and there are ways to be better. To achieve your goals you've got to work at it; you've got to be on a mission, and the mission is one that will never end. It won't be easy. It's not supposed to be. But at the end of the day it's up to you. This is true of everything: picking out which movie to see or what kind of haircut you want to get; deciding how to raise your kids or how hard you're going to work at your job.

Fitness is the same.

You have choices to make—some tough, some easy. You've just got to do it.

You've got to make the decision.

Now go get started.

Be your own hero.

Acknowledgments

I'd like to thank my editor, Michael Homler, for making this happen. Without you this doesn't exist. Also, thanks to Dr. Igal Zuravicky for his added assistance. And as always, thank you to Jack.

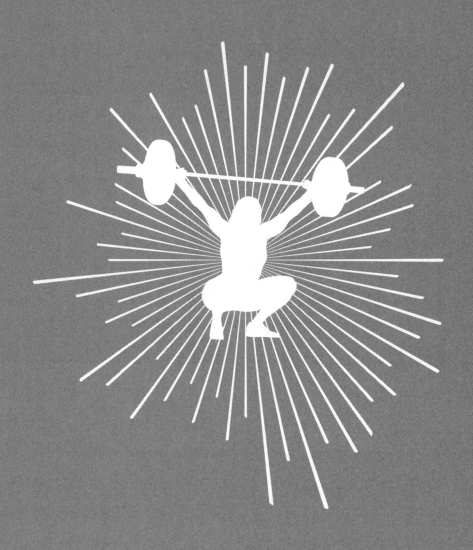

Index

About the Author

DUFFY GAVER is a former Marine sniper and former Navy SEAL. He has trained some of the best actors and actresses Hollywood has to offer for more than twenty years. He also enjoys working as a stuntman and racing motorcycles. He lives in California.

ABOUT THE MODELS

MIKE RYAN is a certified personal trainer. He has trained corporate CEOs, professional athletes, and celebrities, and authored numerous articles on training and fitness. Presently, he resides in Venice, California, and trains every day at Gold's Gym in Venice. Instagram: Mike_ryan_celebrity trainer.

ERIN BROWN is a personal trainer in San Diego with an emphasis in Strength and Conditioning and Nutrition. She is a former Division I athlete and competitive bodybuilder.